COPING WITH YOUR PREMATURE BABY

DR PENNY STANWAY

D1078768

ORION

An Orion Paperback
First published in Great Britain in 1999 by Orion Books Ltd,
Orion House, 5 Upper St Martin's Lane, London WC2H 9EA.

A CIP catalogue record for this book
is available from the British Library.

ISBN: 0 75281 596 2

Printed and bound in Great Britain by
The Guernsey Press Co. Ltd, Guernsey, C.I.

CONTENTS

INTRODUCTION

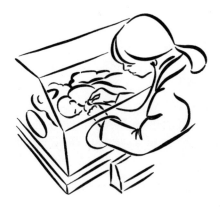

Low-birthweight babies – born too soon or too small – are vulnerable because they aren't fully prepared to face the challenge of life after birth. Extra care boosts their resilience and, particularly for the smallest, their chances of survival itself. And such care is improving all the time.

THE PAST

People haven't always tried to keep very small babies alive. In ancient Rome and Greece many died from a lack of nourishment and warmth, and some were killed outright. The tiniest had little hope of survival then anyway. But philosophers such as Aristotle and Plato held that newborns weren't yet aware of their own existence and therefore weren't fully human – so it didn't much matter whether they lived or died!

Things changed when the Roman Emperor Constantine followed his wife's lead and became a Christian. He then did an about-turn and decreed that his people follow the Judaeo-Christian practice of caring for very small babies because they were human and formed in the image of God.

However, down the ages there have been continued reports of small babies being left to die – some unwanted because they were considered imperfect; others abandoned because they were so unlikely to survive.

THE PRESENT

Today, even with the best of care, it's sometimes clear that a tiny newborn won't pull through. For the fact is that the lower the birthweight, the more hazardous are the early weeks, though modern intensive care is now saving ever smaller and more immature babies.

THE FUTURE

One of the greatest challenges to public health today is to improve women's health and antenatal care, so as to help unborn babies grow big enough to survive and thrive, and make low birthweight less likely.

But the influences on birthweight are complex (see Chapters 16 and 17) and we'll meet this challenge only if everyone – governments, employers, health-care professionals, community groups, families, friends, neighbours, mothers and fathers – works together.

MY EXPERIENCE

Apart from a specialist training in child development and a long-term professional interest, I also have a personal interest. I was a low-birthweight baby myself. I'm lucky enough to have three children now, but I had high blood pressure in each of four pregnancies. When expecting my second daughter I went into premature labour at about 28 weeks; this settled with rest and drug treatment in hospital and she was eventually born three weeks early. And my third baby, a boy, was stillborn at 27 weeks for no apparent reason, though I had fallen down the last four stairs three weeks before while wearing socks; I'd also had a flu-like illness; I'd continued humping furniture around at a weekly parent and toddler group I then ran; and, foolishly, I had tried to restrict my weight gain with a low-calorie diet so as to lower my blood pressure.

I know that some experts consider it wrong to make women believe they can influence whether or not they have a low-birthweight baby. But I disagree. I think many women want to know about anything, however small, that they can do to improve their baby's chances.

And I hope that some of the things I've learnt in the intervening years will help other women look after themselves as well as possible before and after pregnancy.

ABOUT THIS BOOK

- This book is primarily for parents, but others involved with low-birthweight babies may also find it useful.
- I refer to babies as 'he' and 'she' in alternating chapters.
- The book launches straight into premature labour and birth, reflecting the experience of many parents for whom early labour is the first indication of anything unusual; if you prefer definitions first, go to Chapter 3.
- There follows information about special care baby units, and then there's a pause to consider some of the medical jargon you'll come across.
- Next come chapters on what your baby and you need in hospital, on challenges, reactions, bringing your baby home, and development and health in childhood and adult life.

- Then I'll consider why some babies are so small, and how you can look after yourself when considering another pregnancy and once actually pregnant again.
- Last, there's a help list of addresses, books and products.

A TEAM EFFORT

Everyone – parents and medical staff alike – wants the best for a small baby and this often calls for a team effort. I hope this book will help as you play your part.

CHAPTER 1
Premature Labour and Birth

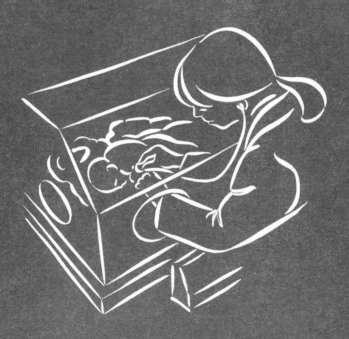

Going into labour unexpectedly early is a shock because you get so used to the idea of having your baby on a particular date. And of course other people do, too.

The question everyone always asks is: 'When's the baby due?' But babies don't always arrive on time and quite a few are premature – born too soon.

SIGNS OF PREMATURE LABOUR

The signs vary, but you may notice:
- Increasingly frequent 'practice' contractions. Put your hand on your tummy and you'll notice your womb tightening and hardening
- Regular contractions
- Increasingly powerful contractions, starting like period pains and becoming more intense
- A trickle or gush of fluid as the amniotic fluid ('waters' or liquor) around the baby escapes
- A few women experience virtually nothing until their baby is nearly out.

WHAT TO DO IF YOU GO INTO LABOUR EARLY

1 **Ring the labour ward**. The staff will probably suggest that you arrange for someone to bring you to hospital at once, or call an ambulance.
2 **Lie down if your waters have broken**. Early in labour a premature baby's head or bottom (the 'presenting part') may not

be positioned well down in the cervix ('engaged' like a stopper in a bottle). If you stay upright, the umbilical cord can readily float downwards into the cervix ('cord prolapse'). Then as your contractions push your baby's presenting part against the cervix, the cord is easily trapped and squashed between the baby and the cervix or vaginal wall. If this blocks the baby's oxygen-carrying blood supply, an emergency Caesarean operation or rapid forceps delivery is essential. Lying down makes the cord less likely to get trapped.

IS IT A FALSE START?

It can be difficult to know whether what you think is labour is the real thing, because only 50 per cent of women who think they're in premature labour actually are. The others find that their

only 50 per cent of women who think they're in premature labour actually are

womb settles within a few hours, though it may be 'jittery' or

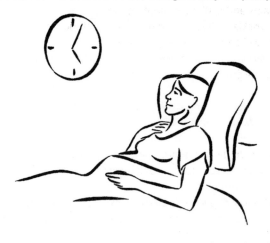

extra-sensitive and contract more than usual for a while, if not for the rest of the pregnancy.

False starts are disruptive and worrying for a woman and her family, and costly in terms of medical care and hospital 'hotel facilities'. As yet there isn't a reliable way of detecting whether labour will progress, but certain things help:

A fetal fibronectin test (see p. 173). If a test for the presence of fetal fibronectin in your vagina is done after 23–24 weeks and the result is negative, you have a 98 per cent chance of not having a premature baby. If the result is positive, you have a one in five chance of labour within four weeks.

Monitoring of womb contractions. A sticky-backed sensor on a woman's abdomen relays the frequency and type of contractions on to screen or paper.

A trans-vaginal ultrasound scan. This detects the shortening, widening and 'funnelling' of the cervix which indicate its 'ripening' (see p. 130) shortly before labour.

CAN AND SHOULD DOCTORS STOP EARLY LABOUR?

If premature labour is well under way, there's very little likelihood of stopping it. But if it's only just begun, there may be some chance.

Whether doctors try depends on several things, including:
• **The length of pregnancy**. They may try to stop labour before 32 weeks because the less mature the baby is, the less likely she is to do well if born early. Between 30 and 32 weeks, her already falling risk of problems from prematurity is reduced even more rapidly
• **The baby's size**. Ultrasound scanning detects whether her size matches the pregnancy dates; some small-for-dates

babies are better out than in; the womb isn't always the best incubator!

- **The baby's state**. Any sign of fetal distress suggests an oxygen shortage, which makes early (perhaps even emergency) delivery wise
- **Your state**. If pregnancy is making you unwell (for example, with worsening pre-eclampsia), it may be sensible to deliver your baby as soon as she stands a reasonable chance, or even – if your life is in jeopardy – as soon as possible. Urine or other infection, diabetes, premature placental separation ('abruption', see p. 136) and placenta praevia (see p. 136) are other possible reasons for not attempting to delay labour
- **Whether the waters have broken**. Once this happens, womb infection is a risk, so it's wise to delay labour only if there's no sign of infection (brown staining of amniotic fluid, an absence of breathing movements by the baby, tender womb and vaginal discharge). Trials currently in progress aim to see if antibiotics can prevent infection and therefore delay labour (see Antibiotics, below). A vaginal swab can reveal the presence of an infection called bacterial vaginosis (see pp. 137 and 151) which can trigger premature labour.

'Late' premature labour – after 35 weeks: One in two premature labours happens between 35 and 37 weeks. Doctors rarely try to prevent these, because if a baby's size matches the dates, she'll be big and mature enough to cope with relatively little help after birth. If the waters have broken but there are no contractions, nature can generally be left to take its course and contractions induced only if there's any trouble.

'Early' premature labour – before 34 weeks: The shorter the pregnancy, the more likely a baby is to need expert help after birth – especially if she's small-for-dates, too. Clearly, it's valuable to try to stop some early labours so the baby can remain in her mother's womb.

However, not every woman needs this intervention, because:

- One in three has a medical reason (such as severe pre-eclampsia) making it best for labour to proceed
- One in three has ruptured membranes – and a risk of getting a womb infection which could harm both mother and baby. However, doctors hope that antibiotics may prevent infection long enough for her baby to stay safely in the womb and grow some more (see Antibiotics, below)
- One in six is already well into labour, with the cervix 3cm or more dilated.

This leaves perhaps only one in six women in labour before 34 weeks who might benefit from having it delayed. And even if it's possible to prolong pregnancy for only a few days, this gives these women time to have the steroid treatment which is so valuable for their babies (see below).

DRUGS WHICH MAY STOP OR DELAY LABOUR

As yet scientists don't know exactly what makes full-term – let alone premature – labour start, but certain drugs can sometimes help prevent the womb expelling the baby early.

These drugs include:

Ritodrine (a beta-agonist) is the most commonly used drug. In one trial this:

- Reduced the chance of premature delivery within 24 hours from over one in four (28 per cent) to around one in ten (11 per cent)
- Reduced the chance of delivery within 48 hours from over one in three (37 per cent) to under one in four (24 per cent).

In another trial, around half the women given drugs delivered within ten days; the other half settled and gave birth only after reaching the safety of 34 weeks. A problem with ritodrine is that it can cause potentially dangerous side effects, especially in those women taking steroids.

Antibiotics. Researchers believe infection with certain bacteria which reach the womb from the vagina may trigger some premature labours.

The Medical Research Council's ORACLE trial is looking at whether certain combinations of antibiotics (amoxycillin and clavulanic acid; or amoxycillin, clavulanic acid and erythromycin) will safely delay labour in women with symptoms of infection who are either in premature labour or whose waters have broken prematurely. This trial also aims to discover whether antibiotics improve a baby's chance of survival or reduce the risk of chronic lung disease and major brain damage.

The PREMET trial aims to discover whether an antibiotic (erythromycin) will help prevent premature labour in women with a raised risk of premature labour because of a positive fetal fibronectin test (see p. 173).

Indomethacin (an anti-prostaglandin and non-steroidal anti-inflammatory drug) is particularly likely to produce side effects, so is generally reserved as a second-line treatment.

Nimesulide is being evaluated and early results look relatively promising.

Glyceryl trinitrate (GTN) skin patches release nitric oxide into the body. Researchers are investigating GTN in the hope that it will relax the womb, widen the placenta's blood vessels, increase the baby's oxygen supply and delay premature labour. However, their early data don't suggest it will be better than ritodrine at delaying premature labour.

TAKING STEROIDS IN PREGNANCY TO HELP YOUR BABY'S BREATHING AFTER BIRTH

After a threatened premature labour, doctors may give a steroid drug (a corticosteroid such as betamethasone) at weekly intervals. This helps the lungs of one in eight babies to grow and mature, improve breathing after birth and makes an oxygen shortage less likely. In turn, this:

- Halves the risk of the respiratory distress syndrome
- Makes necrotising enterocolitis much less likely
- Makes bleeding in the brain much less likely
- Reduces the baby's hospital stay
- Increases the baby's chance of surviving.

INDUCING LABOUR EARLY

Some women have labour induced early for their safety or their baby's.

Reasons for early induction include:

- Illness in the mother (such as diabetes or worsening pre-eclampsia)
- Severe rhesus disease in the baby
- Womb infection
- 'Fetal distress' caused by a lack of oxygen from an unhealthy placenta
- Poor fetal growth, which makes a baby small-for-dates (see p. 27).

Doctors may plan to induce labour early, or may have to induce labour as a semi-emergency. They never decide on it lightly, but carefully consider the baby's maturity, the risk of premature birth and a fight for life outside the womb and, depending on the problem, whether it might be better for the baby to be born early or the mother to be free from her unborn baby.

DELIVERY BY A CAESAREAN OPERATION

It's occasionally best for a baby to be delivered by a Caesarean operation. When planned ahead of time this is called an 'elective' Caesarean.

An emergency Caesarean may be necessary if a premature labour isn't going smoothly or fast enough. And sometimes doctors carry out an emergency Caesarean before a woman goes into labour for her sake or her baby's.

IS PREMATURE LABOUR DIFFERENT FROM ANY OTHER?

There are five main differences between the average premature and full-term labour:

1 **A premature labour leads to a highly charged atmosphere in the labour room**. There's an air of 'alert anxiety' which is good in one sense, as the baby is more likely to need medical attention. However, in another sense it's a pity because tension mars a mother's and father's excitement and awe during the delivery of their child. And a high stress level can make medical intervention more likely (see below).

2 **A premature labour means you need special care, consideration and comfort**. Concern for the baby's well-being is best tempered with calmness and attention to the woman's needs and comfort. In a premature labour, almost more than any other, a woman does best if she's as comfortable as possible. Breathing exercises can help, as can light massage at the base of her spine, an attractive, woman-friendly environment, and other aids to relaxation and pain relief.

3 **A premature labour may make labouring upright particularly important**. Labouring upright in a kneeling or semi-squatting position, rather than lying down, may make labour smoother, easier and quicker. This can reduce the risk of a baby going short of oxygen, and make a forceps or

Caesarean delivery less likely.

However, an upright position isn't always suitable. For example, your obstetrician may advise against it if your waters have broken but the baby's head isn't engaged (see p. 3). If your baby needs continuous fetal monitoring, the monitoring equipment may be of a type which doesn't enable you to leave – or move around on – the bed or delivery table. And some obstetricians are unfamiliar and therefore uneasy with assisting women labouring upright.

In the **first** stage of labour, as the cervix dilates, being upright can encourage smooth, even dilatation of the cervix and effective contractions.

In the **second** stage, as your baby comes out of the womb, being upright can make it easier to adjust your position and to do so frequently. A small change in position can create a big change (30 per cent) in the size of your pelvic outlet. So adjusting your position can give your baby either more room to come out, which can speed delivery and make giving birth less painful, or less room to come out, which can slow delivery if you wish, or if the doctor or midwife recommends it.

When labouring upright you can:

- Walk around (only in the first stage)
- Kneel upright
- Kneel upright with hips bent
- Kneel and bend forwards, holding on to a bed-rail or, if on the floor, some heavy furniture
- Be on all-fours
- 'Semi-squat' – squat with knees and hips somewhat bent, your body upright and, perhaps, someone standing behind and supporting you under the armpits
- Do a full squat, which encourages a much more rapid birth. If you're supple enough for this, you or your attendant must carefully control the baby's birth (see below) because an uncontrolled rapid birth can increase the risk of a bleed into

a premature baby's brain.

- Use a birthing stool, which enables a position roughly equivalent to a semi-squat
- Use a birthing bed – the least favourable option because it tilts a woman's upper body backwards and doesn't allow her to enlarge her pelvic outlet as much as she could.

It isn't good news for a premature baby to rush out in an uncontrolled way. If the midwife or doctor thinks the baby is coming too quickly, you can help control her descent in three ways. First, breathe with little breaths from the top of your chest. Second, put a hand on her head or bottom and press firmly to enable her to emerge more smoothly and slowly. (The midwife or doctor can do this if you prefer.) Third, shift into a less upright position, for example:

- If kneeling upright, bend forward at the hips and hold on to something
- If kneeling, leaning forward and holding on to something, go down on all-fours
- If semi-squatting, stand up more so you're semi-standing
- If semi-squatting or semi-standing, lean forward and hold on to something.

You can use these options to rest more comfortably between contractions, too.

4 **A _premature labour makes sophisticated monitoring more likely._**
This could include:

- Electronic monitoring of the baby's heartbeat (cardiotocography) – either with an ultrasound transmitter strapped to the mother's abdomen, or with a sensor attached to the baby's head or bottom – for signs of fetal distress due to insufficient oxygen
- Measuring the baby's blood gas levels in samples from a scalp vein
- Infra-red scanning to detect oxygen lack before the waters have broken. This method is under evaluation and not

widely available. Researchers shine infra-red and red light through the baby's head with a sensor resting on the baby's cheek. Red, oxygen-rich blood absorbs a different amount of light from blue, oxygen-poor blood. Computer analysis of the light coming through the head indicates any shortage of oxygen. This can also be done after the birth (see p. 96).

5 **A premature labour makes medical intervention more likely.** A doctor may have to intervene to help a distressed baby out of the womb quickly. This can be done by:

• Inducing labour (see above)
• Episiotomy (a cut to widen the vaginal opening)
• Forceps delivery
• Vacuum (ventouse) delivery (only if the cervix is widely enough dilated)
• Emergency Caesarean.

WHEN YOUR BABY ARRIVES

Immediately after delivery, a nurse will lay your baby under a heater. A paediatrician will rapidly assess her condition and give her immediate help if she doesn't start breathing properly. The nurse will dry her, attach an identity tag and wrap her up. In some hospitals a footprint is taken.

Babies younger than 34 weeks need round-the-clock monitoring and treatment in a special care baby unit (SCBU).

Babies of 35–37 weeks need observation and as long as they don't need special or intensive care may be able to go to a 'transitional care' ward with their mothers. Some go to the SCBU, though they may stay with their mothers for a cuddle first. Some are sufficiently well to go to an ordinary postnatal ward with their mothers.

If your baby's blood group is rhesus-positive and yours rhesus-negative, you'll have an injection of anti-D immunoglobulin – antibodies to prevent rhesus disease (which can, at worst, cause stillbirth and the premature birth of a seriously ill baby) in any subsequent rhesus-positive babies you have.

HOW YOU FEEL

Every premature labour and every baby is different and women and their partners react very differently, both at the time and later – see Chapter 12.

TRANSFER TO ANOTHER HOSPITAL

A few very immature, small or unwell babies are transferred by ambulance to an intensive care SCBU at a regional hospital. When a baby is older and fitter she may return to the original hospital closer to home.

Now for some information and tips for coping if your baby needs special care.

CHAPTER 2

The Special Care
Baby Unit

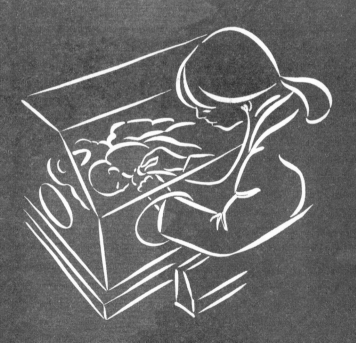

Being suddenly parted from your newborn when he goes off for special or intensive care is tough.

But you know your baby is in skilled hands. And the staff are well aware that you are your baby's most important asset and that you need information and support.

Bigger prems (as premature babies are known in Britain; the North American nickname is 'preemie') may need special care with observation and monitoring of breathing and feeding. Smaller or less mature or healthy babies may need high dependency care, with monitoring and oxygen treatment. Those least able to fend for themselves need intensive care, with monitoring and ventilation.

Nearly every maternity unit in Britain has a special care baby unit (SCBU or 'scaboo'), making a total of 256. Some of these supply intensive care and are known as neonatal intensive care units (NICUs). I'll usually refer to them as SCBUs to save space.

> **Not all SCBU babies are premature or low-birthweight**

Not all SCBU babies are premature or low-birthweight; around half are full-term and have problems such as jaundice or feeding difficulty.

WHAT ABOUT YOU?

After labour and any necessary stitching, washing, tests and checks, most women go to a postnatal ward bed, because only a few SCBUs currently have beds for mothers – or fathers – to sleep near their babies. But you can visit your baby as much as you like. And some SCBUs have a parents' room for relaxing, making drinks and chatting.

If you're too weak or unwell to visit – for example, after a Caesarean – a nurse can bring you a Polaroid photo of your baby. A few SCBUs have closed-circuit TV (CCTV) which enables a mother in the postnatal ward to see her baby on television. And some babies are well enough to be in an incubator by their mothers.

FIRST IMPRESSIONS

Of course, SCBUs do a wonderful job, but they look as alien as the inside of a space capsule. They also smell of hospitals, are very hot and may have harsh, bright fluorescent light. The good news is that the more familiar you become with the environment, equipment and staff, the more settled you'll feel.

SCBU STAFF

The nurses in the SCBU are neonatal nurses of various grades. The doctors may include a senior house officer, and a registrar and consultant who specialise in paediatrics. In teaching hospitals the consultant may be a professor. Nursery nurses help with certain tasks, and specialist staff – such as an audiologist to test hearing and an ophthalmologist to test eyesight – may visit. And there'll be a cleaner and a technician to tend the equipment.

EQUIPMENT

The equipment in an SCBU can help with breathing, oxygen supply, temperature maintenance and feeding. It isn't designed to be parent-friendly, but don't let it frighten you or put you off being with your baby – just see it for what it is, a set of tools.

The staff will use some or all of these tools to help your baby become strong, mature and well enough to go home as soon as possible. If you learn what each item does and what connects with what, everything will rapidly become less intrusive in your relationship with your baby.

First, let's look at your baby's bed.

INCUBATOR

This is a transparent plastic box on wheels. Some have a lid, porthole-like doors and double-glazed walls to retain heat. The air temperature, oxygen level and humidity can be regulated. A fabric cover can keep out the light if necessary.

An open incubator or intensive care cot has no lid, though a heat shield of some sort keeps in the heat when necessary. There may be a stand at one end with shelves, a hanger and an overhead canopy with a radiant heater which can make it into a 'hot cot'.

Beneath the incubator is a cupboard for your baby's nappies, cotton wool, clothes and other things.

KEEPING WARM

A skin temperature sensor can be stuck to a baby's abdomen. This automatically regulates the incubator temperature and sounds an alarm if it gets too hot or cold.

CLEARING HIS THROAT AND MOUTH

The staff use a suction tube to clear mucus or regurgitated milk from a baby's mouth or throat.

FEEDING

A baby who can feed by mouth but not yet by cup, breast

or bottle, is fed through a fine plastic feeding tube (naso-gastric or oro-gastric tube) passed through the nose or mouth, down the gullet and into the stomach. Occasionally, for very premature or unwell babies the feeding tube may be pushed further into the jejunum, so a full stomach can't press on the heart and lungs. The free end is taped to the cheek.

A baby who can't digest food is given liquid feed via a fine plastic IV (intravenous) line (tube or catheter). This enters a vein in the arm, leg, scalp or umbilical cord. An arm or leg line is secured to the limb with tape and a rigid splint prevents the limb moving and dislodging it.

HEART RATE, BREATHING RATE AND BLOOD PRESSURE

The heart rate can be monitored by a sensor stuck to his chest.

The breathing rate can be monitored by a sensor stuck to his chest or abdomen, or a pad placed on the mattress. An alarm sounds if your baby stops breathing, or if his breathing rate or heart rate goes outside pre-set limits. False alarms – usually from a sensor coming unstuck – are common. The breathing centre in the brain which makes a mature baby breathe automatically may not be reliable in a premature one. This can lead to apnoea – 'stop-breathing' – attacks, in which the baby stops breathing for 15–20 seconds. These are best interrupted because they reduce his oxygen supply.

The blood pressure is measured with a tiny arm cuff or, if the baby has an arterial line (catheter), with a monitor attached to this line.

Information about the heartbeat, blood pressure, oxygen level, temperature and breathing pattern are sometimes displayed together on a TV screen.

MONITORING HIS OXYGEN LEVEL

A baby's all-important oxygen level (sometimes called oxygen saturation) depends on several factors, including:

- The oxygen concentration in the air breathed
- His breathing rate
- The maturity and health of his lungs
- His heart rate
- Stress
- Feeds – he uses more oxygen for 15–45 minutes after a feed.

Measurements of 'blood gases' – the amounts of oxygen and carbon dioxide in the blood – are important for babies with a breathing difficulty and can be done in several ways:

A *blood gas analyser* measures oxygen and carbon dioxide in samples taken from an arterial line – a fine tube usually inserted in an artery in the umbilicus, wrist or ankle. Sometimes a tiny arterial sensor in an arterial line monitors the oxygen level directly. (Blood gases may also be measured in blood samples taken from a heel prick, see below.)

A *pulse oximeter* (oxygen saturation monitor) has a light-activated sensor which responds to infra-red light shone through the skin. This registers whether the blood in the skin is red and oxygen-rich or blue and oxygen-poor. If a baby isn't getting enough oxygen, blood leaves the skin for more important organs, so a shortage shows here first. If the oxygen level falls too low, an alarm sounds.

A *transcutaneous monitor* has a heat-activated sensor which measures oxygen and carbon dioxide levels in the blood flowing through a small patch of warmed skin.

HELP WITH BREATHING

1 **Oxygen-rich air** suits babies who can breathe unaided but need extra oxygen. This is either ducted simply into the incubator or into a Perspex head box over the baby's head, or blown through a fine plastic tube opening below the baby's nose. The staff can vary both oxygen concentration and air flow.

2 **A *pressurised flow of oxygen-rich air*** suits babies who need a little help to breathe, as it tops up their oxygen level and keeps their airways open. It's useful, for example, for a very premature baby who gets overtired by breathing, or for one just off a ventilator. The air comes from a continuous positive airway pressure (CPAP) device; it is moistened by a humidifer and delivered through nasal prongs (cannulae) – silicone tubes placed just under or in the nostrils. The staff can vary the oxygen, pressure and humidity levels.

3 **A *mechanical ventilator*** (respirator) 'breathes' for the baby who is too immature or unwell to breathe independently or effectively by pushing oxygen-rich air into his lungs. Common reasons are respiratory distress syndrome and recurrent 'stop-breathing' (apnoea) attacks.

There are two sorts of mechanical ventilator:

* One that does all the breathing, in which case the baby is usually sedated
* One supplying 'baby-triggered ventilation'. Here the baby is able to breathe independently if he can, which is beneficial; but if he misses a beat or doesn't breathe deeply enough, the ventilator breathes for him or boosts his weak breaths.

A ventilator pushes air through wide, ribbed tubing into a plastic endo-tracheal tube which goes through the nose or mouth into the windpipe (trachea). It provides a background stream of slightly pressurised, moist, oxygen-rich air with regular pulses – or breaths – which further inflate the lungs.

After each pulse the lungs deflate somewhat and carbon dioxide escapes. The staff set the ventilator to 'breathe' at 20–40 pulses a minute, and you can hear a click with each one.

Some units use high-frequency ventilation for some babies. This puffs tiny amounts of air into the lungs very rapidly; and if a gadget called an oscillator is also used, it makes the baby's chest vibrate.

The staff aim to get a baby off a ventilator as soon as possible, but it isn't unusual for small prems to go on and off several times before managing on their own permanently.

If a baby has been on a ventilator some time but still can't breathe well enough without it to maintain a satisfactory oxygen level, the doctors may insert a tracheostomy tube through his neck into the windpipe. This leaves the mouth and nose free and can come out when he can breathe unaided.

TREATMENT FOR JAUNDICE

A phototherapy unit is used to shine bright blue or blue-green light (not ultra-violet light) on to a jaundiced baby (see p. 100). It may be a separate piece of equipment or incorporated into the canopy of an open intensive care cot. Eye pads, an eye shield or an orange head shield are used to protect the baby's eyes.

A bilirubinometer is a gadget which measures the level of bilirubin (see p. 100) in a jaundiced baby's serum. This serum is the fluid part of the blood and it is separated from his blood by spinning a blood sample in a centrifuge.

BLOOD TESTS

Some babies need tests for blood gases, haemoglobin, platelets, bilirubin and sugar.

Some premature babies find it hard to regulate their blood sugar level. Low blood sugar (hypoglycaemia) makes them 'jittery' and easily startled. Untreated this can, at worst, lead to convulsions and brain damage. Regular blood sugar tests, perhaps hourly for very small or sick babies, and done on blood taken from a heel-prick, or an IV or arterial line if there is one, alert staff if the level falls too low.

All babies receive blood screening tests. On about the sixth day, a nurse either pricks the baby's heel or takes a blood sample from an IV line, and puts a drop of blood on a 'Guthrie card'. The dried blood spot is tested to see if he has an underactive thyroid gland (congenital hypothyroidism – affecting one in 3000 babies) or phenylketonuria (a condition affecting one in 13,000 babies in which a missing enzyme signals the need for a diet free from the amino acid phenylalanine).

There may soon be routine screening of the same drop of blood for 15 other metabolic conditions.

OTHER INVESTIGATIONS

Regular ultrasound scans of a baby's head – every week, or more often if necessary – give early warning of problems such as bleeding, bruising or scarring in the brain.

All babies receive blood screening tests

X-rays can be used to check that tubes are in the right place, to monitor lung development and to investigate problems.

Researchers are looking at the benefits of repeated infra-red scans of the brain (see p. 96), using a special head visor, to spot early signs of damage.

COSTS

Some pieces of SCBU equipment cost over £30,000. Nursing and medical care are expensive, too, with several health authorities suggesting that a day's care for one baby costs around £500. Other figures indicate that the cost of caring for premature babies weighing less than 1350g (3lb) in the UK each year is up to £70 million. Charities such as Bliss (see p. 176) donate an average of two-thirds of the equipment. Sadly, though, many units remain under-resourced.

HOW YOU MAY FEEL

The first sight of their baby in an incubator pulls every parent's heartstrings. For there, connected, perhaps, to tubes, monitors and other equipment, is the tiny scrap of humanity that just a short time ago was inside his mother's body.

Relief at knowing your labour is over and your baby alive contends with fatigue and a welter of emotions, though some parents feel so drained or shocked they can't feel anything much.

Most SCBU staff are well schooled in helping parents recognise and talk about their feelings. Allowing yourself to do this will help you cope (see Chapter 12).

Now your baby has arrived and you've begun to familiarise yourself with the SCBU, let's look at what prematurity means.

CHAPTER 3

What is Prematurity?

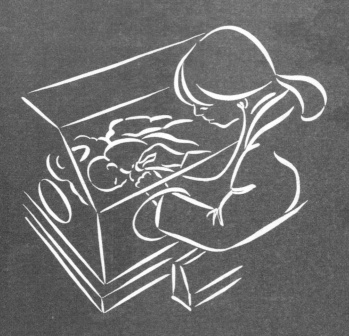

A premature baby is one born before 37 weeks, which doesn't give her enough time in the womb to grow and mature fully.

Nearly all premature babies have a low birthweight and some are also smaller than expected for the length of pregnancy.

HOW LONG IS A NORMAL PREGNANCY?

A normal pregnancy can last anything between 37 and 42 weeks, but an average pregnancy is said to last 40 weeks from the first day of the last period. This isn't accurate, though, because pregnancy begins at conception, which generally occurs around ovulation (day 14 of the average cycle). So the first day of the last period is simply a convenient point from which to date pregnancy, and some unborn babies and newborns are two weeks younger than the due date suggests.

A premature baby is one born before 37 weeks

WORKING OUT YOUR DUE DATE

There are three steps:
1 Take the date of the first day of your last period.
2 Count forward nine calendar months (March, April, May and so on, not four-week lunar months).
3 Add one week.

However, while nine out of ten babies are born within two weeks of the due date, only seven in 100 arrive on the day itself!

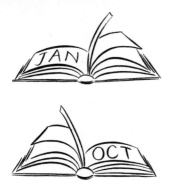

while nine out of ten babies are born within two weeks of the due date, only seven in 100 arrive on the day itself

FULL-TERM AND PREMATURE (PRE-TERM) BABIES

Babies born between 37 and 42 weeks are described as full-term, while those born before 37 weeks are premature. But astonishingly, the Department of Health currently doesn't collect the figures indicating how many babies are born prematurely.

A rough estimate is that between five and seven per cent of the babies born in England and Wales each year are premature. Taking the 642,100 babies born in 1997 as an example, this would mean that roughly between 32,000 and 45,000 were premature.

Around 18,000 of these babies were very premature – born before 34 weeks – and around 6000 extremely premature – born before 30 weeks.

SMALL-FOR-DATES, SMALL-FOR-GESTATIONAL-AGE, OR GROWTH-RETARDED BABIES

A baby's gestational age is the same as the length of pregnancy.

The weight of 'small-for-dates' or 'small-for-gestational-age' babies is inappropriate for their gestational age, meaning they are lighter, shorter and thinner than normal for that length of pregnancy.

One baby in ten suffers from growth-retardation (intra-uterine growth-retardation or IUGR) in the womb and is born relatively small-for-dates. And some growth-retarded babies are much lighter than others of a similar gestational age. A growth-retarded baby may have more difficulty with breathing, feeding and illness than a baby of the same gestational age whose weight is appropriate for the length of pregnancy.

HOW MUCH DO NEWBORNS WEIGH?

A healthy, full-term newborn generally weighs from 2500g (5lb 8oz) to 4500g (9lb 14oz). The average birthweight is slowly rising over the years and is now 3320g (7lb 5oz).

average birthweight is slowly rising

You may find this conversion chart helpful:

Metric	Imperial
500g	1lb 2oz
750g	1lb 10oz
1000g	2lb 3oz
1250g	2lb 12oz
1500g	3lb 5oz
1750g	3lb 14oz
2000g	4lb 6oz
2250g	4lb 15oz
2500g	5lb 8oz

LOW-BIRTHWEIGHT BABIES – PRE-MATURE, SMALL-FOR-DATES OR BOTH?

A low birthweight is defined as less than 2500g (5lb 8oz); the UK has one of the highest proportions of low-birthweight babies in Europe.

In 1997 there were 642,100 live-born babies in England and Wales. Of these, 47,742 – that's 7.4 per cent, or one in 13 – weighed less than 2500g. A comparison of the women in 12 European countries reveals that the English and Welsh have the third highest risk of having a low-birthweight baby after the Hungarians and Poles. Scots women have the fourth highest risk, but that of women in the Irish Republic is second to lowest.

What's more, 7873 babies in England and Wales – that's 1.2 per cent, or one in 81 – weighed less than 1500g (3lb 5oz).

A baby's birthweight may be low because she is:

- Premature. Two out of three low-birthweight babies are premature – in 1996 in England and Wales over 31,000 premature babies were born
- Small-for-dates. One in three low-birthweight babies is born over 37 weeks
- Both premature and small-for-dates.

Very low birthweight is defined as less than 1500g (3lb 5oz). A birthweight of 1500g – about the same as a big bag of flour – is appropriate for a gestational age of 32–34 weeks.

Extremely low birthweight is usually defined as less than 1000g. A birthweight of around 500g – about the same as a small bag of sugar – is appropriate for a gestational age of 23–24 weeks.

MISCARRIAGE AND STILLBIRTH

A miscarriage is now defined as the ending of pregnancy before 24 weeks. One in every two or three pregnancies probably ends this way. A stillbirth is now defined as the delivery of a dead baby after 24 weeks.

Anything that damages a pregnant woman and harms her baby makes miscarriage and stillbirth more likely. Such things include:

- A poor diet
- Being seriously under- or overweight
- Too much alcohol
- Smoking
- Shock
- Poisoning from pesticides, fumes from burning plastic, X-rays, fumes or dust from stripping lead paint, vapour from solvents and glues, and certain industrial chemicals
- Infections such as chickenpox, rubella (German measles) and flu (viral infections); toxoplasmosis (an infection with tiny organisms called protozoa) and listeriosis (a bacterial infection)
- Vaccines containing live viruses (for example, polio and yellow fever).

These very same things also prevent some couples conceiving and make both premature birth (see Chapter 15) and stillbirth more likely. I think we might learn more about preventing fertility problems, miscarriage, stillbirth and prematurity if we looked at them as different outcomes of the same triggers.

The next thing to consider is what your premature baby needs.

CHAPTER 4

What Your Baby Needs

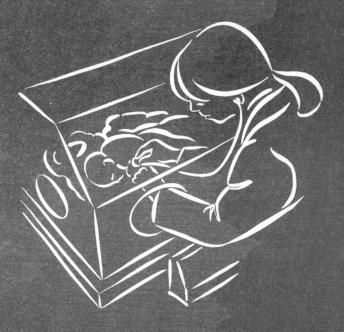

L ike all babies, premature and other low-birthweight ones need nourishment, protection, care and human contact.

Most important, your baby needs love – one-to-one attention from people with his well-being at heart. You and your partner can probably supply this better than anyone else, though the nurses will do what they can. So if he needs special care, one of you should try to stay with him as much as possible. Given the opportunity, a small baby soon learns to recognise his mother and father, and if mature and well enough, he may show this recognition by being calm or excited, or meeting their gaze.

a small baby soon learns to recognise his mother and father

Your baby is an individual. You'll gradually learn his likes and dislikes, what stresses and calms him, and how much he sleeps. And you can help the staff as he grows, develops, and gets out of his incubator and home as soon as possible.

WHAT HE NEEDS

It helps to think of your baby's age in terms of 'post-conception' age – the length of pregnancy plus the time since birth. The lower this is, the more skilled care he'll probably need.

Premature babies may be:

EXTREMELY PREMATURE: 24–29 WEEKS POST-CONCEPTION AGE

These need:
- Incubator care
- Monitoring
- IV- or tube-feeding
- Special skin care
- Help with breathing (ventilation, CPAP or extra oxygen). Most very-low-birthweight babies (less than 1500g) need extra oxygen; one in two needs CPAP or ventilation; and one in ten goes home on extra oxygen.

VERY PREMATURE: 30–34 WEEKS POST-CONCEPTION AGE

These mostly have a low birthweight and need:
- Incubator care
- Monitoring
- Tube- or cup-feeding plus practice at the breast (or bottle)
- Help with breathing (usually CPAP or extra oxygen; some need ventilation) until they breathe unaided. Most of those whose birthweight is very low (less than 1500g) need extra oxygen; one in two needs CPAP or ventilation; one in ten goes home on extra oxygen.

PREMATURE: 35–37 WEEKS POST-CONCEPTION AGE

These may have a low birthweight and need:
- Adequate warmth
- Monitoring – usually for a few days at least
- Patience while learning to breastfeed (or bottle-feed); cup-feeding if necessary
- Help with breathing for the few who can't yet breathe unaided (usually extra oxygen, and occasionally CPAP or even ventilation). Needing help with breathing is especially

common after a Caesarean, because such a baby has bene-fited neither from the surge of maternal stress hormones during labour, nor from the womb contractions which would have emptied fluid from his lungs.

IN THE INCUBATOR

POSITION

The staff may lay your baby on his tummy to encourage better breathing and sleeping and to discourage movement to save energy. The 'Back to Sleep' campaign recom-mends reducing the risk of sudden infant death by putting babies on their backs to sleep (see p. 114). You needn't be concerned about your baby being on his tummy because the staff will observe him and breathing and heart monitors give added peace of mind.

> *Babies feel calmer and grow better when well sup-ported and semi-cocooned.*

Your baby may need his position changed frequently, and the mattress may be tilted to raise his head and to aid diges-tion and breathing.

Babies feel calmer and grow better when well supported and semi-cocooned. This helps them feel comfortable and 'contained'. Possibilities include a specially shaped fabric or foam roll, wedge, bolster, pillow or nest. Some SCBUs cushion a baby's head with a beanbag to prevent it being flattened.

Many small babies stay in an incubator until around 34 weeks post-conception age or until they weigh 1350–1800g (3–4lb).

KEEPING WARM

A premature baby's temperature-regulating mechanisms aren't mature and he can't shiver or sweat. He hasn't enough fat to keep him warm, because fat appears beneath the skin only in the last few weeks of full-term pregnancy. And he lacks 'brown fat' – a type of fat which is a ready source of heat energy and found in full-terms between the shoulder blades and around the kidneys.

Small-for-dates babies lack body fat and easily get cold, too.

An incubator provides a constant temperature and a radiant heater can supply extra heat. Small babies also stay warm if nursed kangaroo-style (see p. 80).

PREVENTING DRY SKIN

An extremely premature baby's skin is very thin so it easily dries and cracks. An incubator's high humidity helps prevent water loss, as does covering the skin. Some units use a liquid paraffin derivative to retain moisture.

SLEEP

Deep sleep helps your baby grow and develop. Quiet times with minimal noise, light and touching help him sleep. Once your baby is able to leave the incubator, you'll find he sleeps better in your arms than in the incubator.

PROTECTION FROM INFECTION

A mother's antibodies don't cross the placenta until 32 weeks, so the immune system of a baby born earlier doesn't protect him very well.

You can help by:
• Providing breast milk
• Avoiding close contact with outsiders
• Washing your hands before touching your baby
• Wearing a mask if you have a cough or cold
• Not touching a cold sore or active genital herpes infection.

PROTECTION FROM BRIGHT LIGHT

The SCBU lighting may be extremely bright. Indeed, 15 minutes of the amount of light recommended by the American Academy of Pediatrics for SCBUs so the staff can see clearly, is over nine times the US industrial safety regulations' limit for healthy adult eyes!

This can be bad news for premature babies because their eyes are particularly vulnerable to bright light. Their eyes stay open more than those of full-term ones, even in bright light. And their thinner eyelids and larger pupils transmit more light.

Bright light prevents very-low-birthweight babies getting enough deep sleep. It can also make them restless, decrease weight gain and reduce their 'islands of wakefulness' (see p. 71). At worst, it may harm their eyes (see p. 99).

You and the staff can help by:
- Keeping background lighting low
- Using dimmer switches to prevent the sudden changes of brightness which make some babies short of oxygen
- Drawing curtains on bright days
- Covering the incubator unless a very ill or small baby needs observation for skin colour changes, difficult breathing, restlessness and other problems
- Covering a head box
- Draping a cover over his head if he's on a ventilator
- Putting goggles on him until a post-conception age of 31 weeks
- Shielding his eyes under a radiant heater
- Screening a phototherapy unit shining on a nearby baby
- Directing extra lighting away from his eyes
- Dimming the light regularly when he reaches a post-conception age of 30–32 weeks
- Having separate lighting controls for each incubator.

PROTECTION FROM NOISE

Loud or sudden sounds stress an immature baby, impair sleep and can reduce his oxygen level. Loud noises may also prevent him from beginning to learn to distinguish speech patterns. An SCBU can be noisy with equipment running, telephones ringing, doors and drawers opening and closing, and people talking. The British Safety Standard for noise in an incubator is 60 decibels maximum, and one American researcher recommends this should be less than 50 decibels. However, sounds of 120 decibels have been recorded in an SCBU – and average peak SCBU noise levels in one US hospital were above 80 decibels (the equivalent of raucous music) – and an incubator gives little protection.

These things help protect your baby:
- Talking quietly
- Having quiet times
- Putting a 'Quiet – baby sleeping' notice on the incubator
- Preventing unnecessary sound, such as from a radio
- Reducing the ringing volume of telephones or replacing a ring with a flashing light
- Not banging doors, drawers and rubbish bins
- Moving equipment quietly
- Tending to crying babies promptly
- Using a padded incubator cover
- Attending to alarms quickly
- Replacing noisy alarms with flashing lights
- Replacing staff bleeps with vibrating radio pagers
- Frequently removing water from ventilator tubing.

YOUR VOICE, HEARTBEAT AND OTHER BODY SOUNDS

Hearing your voice and listening to your heartbeat, tummy rumbles and other body sounds is comforting and soothing to your baby. If you or your partner can't be there, you could make a tape of your voices.

YOUR SMELL

Recognising your natural scent may relax your baby and is particularly important when he's learning to breastfeed (see p. 72). And just putting one of your used breast pads by him in the incubator may help him relax.

TOUCH

Small babies who are stroked and cuddled grow and develop quicker. A study of healthy pre-terms of less than 36 weeks post-conception age showed that stroking and other touching increased their weight gain by 47 per cent a day! A similar study found extra touching enabled prems

to go home sooner. Stroking can interrupt 'stop-breathing' (apnoea) attacks, and letting your baby hold your finger may calm him and help him breathe.

There's no touch so welcome as that of a loving parent, and the rewards are mutual. Colombian researchers found fewer mothers abandoned premature babies if they touched and held them. If you're not there, it's important for someone else to touch your baby.

If your baby is very premature or ill, the nurses may suggest touching him as little as possible to prevent bruising him or disturbing his sleep.

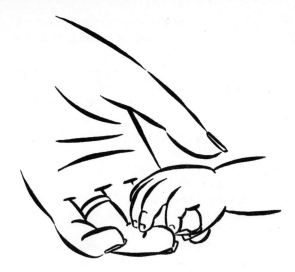

When something has to be done, he'll have less of a shock if you rouse him first by:
- Stroking him gently
- Giving him a finger to hold
- Letting him suck a (clean) fingertip or dummy
- Wrapping him in a blanket
- Slowly raising the light level
- Talking or singing softly.

Some babies are less stressed if essential procedures are grouped together, though the most unwell and immature may do better if they recover after each one.

Gently cupping the top of his head with one hand and laying the other on his back may comfort him.

As *your baby grows and develops or becomes healthier*, you'll be able to touch him more. Indeed, a baby of 28 weeks post-conception age will probably manage an hour of actual cuddling. He'll probably love being massaged and may sleep well and need less oxygen afterwards. Keep him warm, turn the lighting down and wash and warm your hands, then use a little warm oil (such as almond oil) and let your hands express your love by moving over his body.

If *your baby doesn't need incubator care*, cuddle and touch him as much as you like.

YOUR BABY'S RESPONSES

Caring for a tiny baby can seem unrewarding, particularly if he isn't yet looking at you and can't be in your arms or at your breast. But learning to recognise how he's feeling can make you feel more involved:

When *he's stressed* he may cry; screw up his eyes; pull a face; go limp; yawn a lot; vomit; not grasp your finger; look bluish, pale, grey or mottled; tremble, twitch or 'jump'; struggle; or breathe irregularly.

When *he's contented* he may look relaxed; sleep deeply; be alert more often; put his hand to his mouth; look at you when you speak; move smoothly; hold or suck your finger; have a good colour; and breathe steadily and easily.

CAN HE FEEL PAIN?

Babies become consciously aware of pain after 26 weeks post-conception age. Before this, they react to pain at a reflex, spinal level, and may flinch when touched or show other signs of stress (see above).

However carefully done, some procedures will hurt, but your baby may suffer less if:

- You or the staff either wait for an 'island of wakefulness' (see p. 71) or wake him gently first (see p. 39)
- You distract him by speaking or stroking gently

• You touch or cuddle him so he's soothed by your proximity and heartbeat.

NAPPY-CHANGING

You may have to supply nappies, creams, cotton wool and other toiletries.

Change your baby's nappy as soon as it's wet or soiled, as a damp nappy quickly cools a small baby. The nurses will show you how to avoid dislodging any tubes and wires. You'll probably feel clumsy at first, but the most experienced person in the SCBU had to start some time and you'll soon become more adept.

CLEANING

Small wet babies rapidly become chilled when washed or cleaned with baby oil, so the nurses may recommend extra heat from a radiant heater. Being washed can be stressful and increase your baby's need for oxygen.

SWADDLING

Many babies like being wrapped firmly – perhaps because they feel more secure. This swaddling encourages them to cry less, sleep more and save energy by moving less. It may also increase their oxygen level.

MOVEMENT

A baby mature and well enough to be out of an incubator is comforted by being rocked, perhaps because it triggers memories of being in the womb. Rocking encourages rhythmic breathing and deep sleep. If you use a sling or carry your baby kangaroo-style (see p. 80), you'll provide motion and warmth.

CLOTHES

A baby may wear only a nappy and a knitted bonnet or other hat in an incubator. A hat is important because a bare head loses so much heat.

Most clothes and nappies are much too big for low-birth-weight babies, and only when they are about 3000g (6lb 10oz) will standard nappies and stretch-suits fit. However, small ones are available (see p. 179).

NAPPIES
You could try the following:
• Double-fold standard muslin nappies
• Make small nappies from terry towelling
• Cut standard terry-towelling nappies diagonally and hem the long edge
• Cut down disposables and tape their raw edges.

WATERPROOF PANTS
Take a first-size pair and sew extra seams to make the leg and waist holes smaller.

Remind friends and relatives you don't want too many tiny clothes. It's better to have bigger ones for your baby to grow into.

TOYS

A premature baby of over 30 weeks post-conception age may enjoy a bright mobile – especially if it is black, white, red or orange. A musical toy might appeal, too. Easily cleaned plastic toys are best as soft toys harbour germs.

So much for what your baby needs after his bumpy start – but what about you?

CHAPTER 5

What You Need

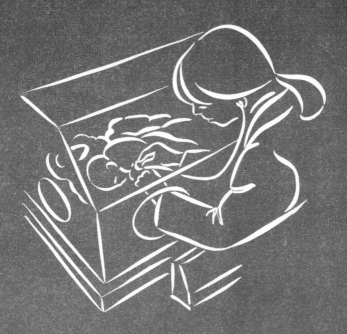

Having a low-birthweight baby is like having a child star. After you've done such a lot to get her where she is, she's the centre of attention and you're left high and dry.

But whether your baby comes straight home or stays in hospital, it's vital for you as parents to think of yourselves and your needs. You are very important people – as

it's vital for you as parents to think of yourselves and your needs

individuals, to one another, and to your baby. So please take the advice in this chapter and build on it. For information about practical issues while your baby is in hospital, turn to Chapter 10. And for help with emotional and other reactions, see Chapter 12.

FOOD AND DRINK

You need the best possible nourishment because:
• After pregnancy you may need to top up on several nutrients
• You need an extra 400–600 calories a day to replace those in breast milk
• You need to fill your milk with nutrients without depleting your body
• Stress may deplete you of certain nutrients.

If you stay in hospital, make sure you eat five helpings a day of fresh vegetables, salads and fruit, even if you have to buy your own or have them brought in. Eat proper meals and nutritious between-meals snacks and reserve biscuits, cakes, sweets, crisps and chocolate from hospital vending machines as occasional treats. And drink plenty of fluid to produce milk and counteract the SCBU's hot, dry atmosphere.

SUPPLEMENTS?

Supplements aren't officially recommended for a healthy woman who's just had a low-birthweight baby, provided she eats a healthy diet and spends some time outside each day.

However, if you're not eating properly, or are closeted inside, and decide to take a food supplement, choose:

If _you're breastfeeding_: a multivitamin and mineral product suitable for nursing mothers, and fish oil to provide extra DHA (docosahexaenoic acid, see p. 51, a fatty acid which aids brain development in pre-term babies). Our bodies usually make plenty of DHA from essential fatty acids in foods, but a top-up won't hurt.

If _you're not breastfeeding_: any multipurpose, multivitamin and mineral product.

Ask your pharmacist if unsure. And if you can't leave hospital, ask a relative or friend to enquire on your behalf.

PROTECTION AGAINST DEVELOPING RHESUS ANTIBODIES

If your blood group is rhesus-negative and your baby's rhesus-positive, then within 72 hours of the birth you'll have an injection of anti-D immunoglobulin antibodies. This destroys any of the baby's blood cells which have leaked into your bloodstream and prevents your immune system setting up an antibody production system which might damage future rhesus-positive babies (see p. 174).

THE RIGHT CLOTHES

Wear light clothes because hospitals are always hot.

When your baby is bigger and stronger, you can pull up a T-shirt or other top for breastfeeding. But it's easier with a very young, small baby if no clothes get in the way, so wear something that undoes in front. If you prefer not to expose your breast, pull up a loose T-shirt and secure the fold of fabric with a clothes peg, hair clip or bulldog clip so it covers most of your breast but leaves the baby's nose and your hands free.

LIGHT

As soon as you can, get outside for at least ten minutes midday, longer at other times, to get daylight on your face. This encourages your body to make vitamin D (for healthy bones), oestrogen, and serotonin (a 'feel-good' chemical).

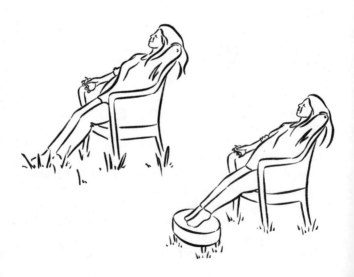

POST-NATAL EXERCISES

The early weeks of mothering a premature baby can be very busy but it's important to make time for post-natal exercises, including pelvic floor exercises. Your midwife or health visitor will advise you.

PRACTICAL HELP

If you need help, ask the staff, visitors or your partner. One ongoing necessity, for example, is coins or phone cards to make calls; you can't use a mobile phone in hospital as it disturbs electronic equipment.

SEX

It's easy to forget contraception when you start having intercourse again. Yet you probably won't want to start another baby while so involved with this one, so it's sensible to take precautions early.

ENCOURAGEMENT AND AFFIRMATION

These magnify the positives in life and make the negatives less important.

For example:

- Focus on anything positive – big or small – in what you're doing and how you're doing it
- Do the same for your partner by warmly describing something positive about what he's doing or how he's doing it
- Focus on any progress your baby is making, however tiny
- However 'fetal' your baby looks, think of something you like about her appearance or behaviour
- At the end of each day, reflect on everything good that's

happened and every kindness shown
- Thank, encourage and affirm members of staff when appropriate
- Do the same to other parents and to supportive friends and relatives.

STRESS-MANAGEMENT

Make time to recognise the signs of stress sooner rather than later. If, as is likely, you can't remove the stress, find ways of looking after yourself.

How about:

- Relaxing with a couple of rests each day, the TV, a book or a leisurely scented bath (yes – even in hospital). And don't forget, laughter is one of the best medicines
- Taking daily exercise as soon as you can
- Keeping a diary. Logging events and feelings can help when living through challenging experiences
- Enjoying the creativity of recording your baby's days by taking photos and describing each one in a photo album, or making a video to look at later.

RIGHTS AND BENEFITS

Check – or ask someone else to check – that you and your family are getting the state and other benefits to which you're entitled.

Now to what your baby needs by way of nourishment.

CHAPTER 6

Nutrition for Small Babies

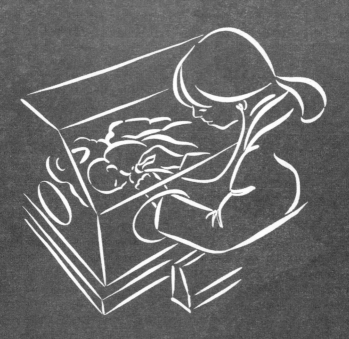

Small babies have special nutritional needs. Prems need more fluid and calories per pound of body weight than do full-terms, and small-for-dates babies have a lot of catching up to do, too.

Small babies can manage only small feeds, partly because digestion uses a lot of their available energy, so they need feeding frequently. They need high quality food for growth and development and to combat infections and stress. And they may need feeding by IV line, tube or cup before they progress to the breast (or bottle).

Prems need more fluid and calories per pound of body weight

First, let's look at your choice of milk.

CHOICE OF MILK

You have three options: breast milk, formula or both.

BREAST MILK
This is the best food for babies old enough to digest milk, and is particularly important for prems. A wonderful thing about your milk is that its composition will change as your baby grows. The few drops of the very first milk – creamy, yellowish-white colostrum – are rich in the very things he most needs, including valuable minerals such as zinc, anti-infective factors (including live cells, enzymes, hormones, lactoferrin and

lysozyme), growth factors and protein. Having colostrum makes a baby less likely to become jaundiced.

The thinner-looking milk which comes next contains 30 per cent more protein than the milk you'll make as your baby nears 40 weeks post-conception age. It also has more of certain minerals (magnesium, phosphorus, sodium and ionised, easy-to-use calcium) and more anti-infective substances (lactoferrin, lysozyme, antibodies – especially immunoglobulin A – and live cells).

Milk fat is well absorbed and provides 50 per cent of the calories he needs. And, most important, it's rich in certain long-chain polyunsaturated fatty acids (also known as LCPs, long-chain PUFAs or LCPUFAs). These – both DHA (docosahexaenoic acid, an omega-3 fatty acid) and AA (arachidonic acid, an omega-6 fatty acid) – are important for brain, eye and nerve development. About a quarter of a baby's brain is made of DHA and AA.

It's particularly important for a premature baby to get plenty of DHA. Such a baby misses out on the large amount of DHA which passes across the placenta in the last weeks of a full-term pregnancy and therefore needs good supplies so the brain can grow rapidly in the first three months after birth.

Fortifying breast milk. After the first four weeks, your milk's protein level will fall. If necessary the paediatrician will recommend fortifying it with protein, vitamins (such as E) and minerals (calcium, copper, iron, phosphorus and zinc) to aid your baby's growth and development.

A breast-milk fortifier may help if your baby is:
- Very small
- Not growing fast enough
- Receiving donated milk (see below)
- Tube-fed – because some fat sticks to the tube and gets lost.

FORMULA

Pre-term formula is better than standard formula for premature babies younger than 34 weeks post-conception age. Manufacturers try to copy pre-term breast milk, which is why they've recently added DHA, but they can't add such things as a mother's live cells and antibodies. Breast milk is best for all babies, premature or otherwise.

> *Manufacturers try to copy pre-term breast milk*

BENEFITS OF BREAST MILK COMPARED WITH FORMULA

Breast milk provably provides the following benefits (those in bold are particularly important for premature babies):

- **The right nutrients in the right proportions for a baby's post-conception age**
- **Better digestion**, particularly of fat and calcium. Breast milk stimulates bowel function, movement, and hormone and enzyme production, and encourages a healthy population of micro-organisms (the 'bowel flora')
- **Good growth rate**, of around the rate a baby would have grown had he stayed in the womb, or a little slower. Small-for-dates babies who are breastfed grow faster in the first year than those who are formula-fed. And in the first three months their heads grow faster, probably reflecting better brain growth
- **Less illness**
- **Fewer infections**, such as pneumonia, gastroenteritis and ear infection
- **Fewer allergic problems**, such as asthma and eczema
- **Lower risk of anaemia**, because iron is better absorbed
- **Reduced risk of meconium ileus** (bowel paralysis, generally

in babies with cystic fibrosis, caused by sticky bowel contents)

- **Reduced risk of necrotising enterocolitis** (see p. 99), a dangerous reaction to a bowel infection which kills up to two in five affected babies, and is six to ten times more common in babies fed on formula alone compared with those fed on breast milk alone. Babies on formula plus breast milk have a lower risk than formula-only babies, but three times the risk of those on breast milk alone
- **Higher development and intelligence test results**
- **Better visual development and eyesight**
- Earlier walking
- A lower risk of young-onset diabetes
- Less dental decay.

And research suggests that breast milk also reduces the risk of:

- **'Stop-breathing' (apnoea) attacks**
- **Convulsions**
- **Unexplained cot death** (see p. 114)
- Coeliac disease (intolerance to gluten, a cereal grain protein)
- Pyloric stenosis (a stomach condition causing vomiting and, perhaps, failure to thrive)
- Appendicitis
- Ulcerative colitis and Crohn's disease (inflammatory bowel diseases)
- Jaw and mouth problems
- Lymphoma (lymph system cancer).

The process of breastfeeding is less stressful to a very small baby than bottle-feeding, and makes it easier to breathe and get enough oxygen. It's also a way of communicating your love and developing your relationship. And it fast becomes an effective way of comforting or relaxing your baby at any time.

What's more, breastfeeding has future health benefits for mothers, too. For example, it will lower your risk of ovary cancer, and of breast cancer before your menopause, and will make hip fractures less likely when you're over 65.

BREAST OR BOTTLE?

Even if you had intended to bottle-feed, please think again, because studies show that bottle-feeders are less aware than other women of the benefits and practicalities of breastfeeding, and it's better to make an informed choice.

For example, many such women wrongly believe breastfeeding will spoil their figures (whereas it's pregnancy, not breastfeeding, that changes breasts). Some think providing milk and breastfeeding will tie them down, be embarrassing or hinder their return to work; they see bottle-feeding as freeing women from having to care for their babies. However, each of these points has strong counter-arguments.

You may want to copy bottle-feeding friends – but why not set a trend yourself? Or you may fear breastfeeding will hurt

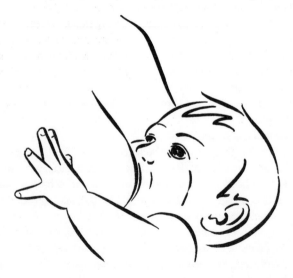

(which it can, though there are almost always solutions). You may feel breastfeeding is unsexy or disgusting (a matter of opinion), or fear failure (which need only rarely happen – *and anyway, a little breast milk is a great deal better than none*). Some women fancy the equipment and rituals of bottle-feeding (and don't realise breastfeeding has its own mystique).

If you share any of these views, please read the suggestions in *Breast is Best* (see p. 179).

CAN MOTHERS OF PREMATURE BABIES MAKE ENOUGH MILK?

Women who deliver early can certainly breastfeed. Indeed, many women report making two or three times as much milk as their small baby needs and enjoy the privilege of donating the excess to a milk bank.

However, making enough milk and breastfeeding a prem can sometimes be difficult, because:

- Expressing or pumping milk is time-consuming and less immediately rewarding than breastfeeding
- The lack of the presence and smell of her baby when he can't leave the incubator removes a powerful stimulus for the milk to be 'let down' (to flow spontaneously)
- The ups and downs of a small baby's progress can be stressful and, at worst, can affect the let-down of breast milk
- The SCBU's stark, clinical, high-tech environment makes some mothers doubt their ability and feel tense and uneasy
- The SCBU may have a bottle-feeding ethos, with staff paying lip-service to the value of breast milk but preferring formula because it's easier not to bother with the expertise, sensitivity and patience needed to inform, encourage and support mothers learning how to provide breast milk. In my view these skills are some of the most important for SCBU doctors and nurses to learn.

Now to the feeding process itself.

IV FEEDING

The smallest (under 1000g – 2lb 3oz) and most unwell babies, including those on a ventilator, have liquid feed via a fine tube into a vein (IV line). At first this contains glucose and salts and later, perhaps, amino acids, vitamins, minerals and fats, too. The IV line is moved frequently to avoid irritating any one vein.

When the nurses think he's ready, he can have a few drops of your colostrum down a feeding tube into his stomach. Colostrum stimulates the production of hormones which help the digestive system to mature. When a baby can digest milk and breathe unaided, he can progress to tube-feeding. When he can take enough by tube, IV feeds are no longer necessary.

TUBE-FEEDING

If a baby's digestive system is ready for oral feeds but he can't yet drink efficiently, he can have milk via a tube into his stomach (or duodenum). Babies are tube-fed if they:
• Are less than 32 weeks post-conception age
• Breathe faster than 75 breaths a minute
• Can't yet co-ordinate sucking, swallowing, breathing and gagging.
One benefit is the lack of effort needed by a baby whose strength is best put into growth and development.

A feed of breast milk (or formula) may be allowed to drip from a syringe down the tube. Feeds are frequent (one hourly to three or four hourly, depending on size and needs) and small. A 900g (2lb) baby, for example, might have only 10–15 ml (2–3 teaspoons) of milk an hour.

Feeds are pushed from the syringe down the tube for some babies. And for others an electric pump continuously propels milk down the tube.

Most babies don't seem to mind the feeding tube remaining

in place between feeds. But if yours objects, a new one can be inserted each time.

You may notice your baby opening and closing his mouth, putting out his tongue or sucking his fingers during a tube-feed. This shows he is ready to practise sucking at the breast.

PRACTICE-SUCKING AT THE BREAST FOR TUBE-FED BABIES

If your baby is well enough to come out of the incubator, give him lots of opportunities to be at your breast so he can enjoy its proximity and one day, when he's mature and interested enough, start licking milk and, eventually, practice-sucking. It's a good idea to have him by the breast while he's receiving a tube-feed (see below).

> *practice-sucking during a tube-feed enhances digestion*

Apart from getting the milk that drips or flows during a let-down or leaks from your full breast, he won't breastfeed 'properly' and take much milk until he's mature enough to suck, 'milk' the breast (see p. 72), and co-ordinate breathing, sucking and swallowing. But although sucking practice is 'non-nutritive', it's important to his digestion, growth and well-being, and boosts your milk supply.

Babies allowed sucking practice (during a tube-feed and at other times) provably have:

1 Higher oxygen levels
2 More alertness before feeds
3 Better weight gain
4 Earlier co-ordination of breathing, sucking and swallowing, allowing them to cup-feed or breastfeed sooner
5 An earlier return home.

One possible explanation for points 3, 4 and 5 is that

practice-sucking during a tube-feed enhances digestion – perhaps by stimulating the vagus nerve which may:

- Decrease the level of the hormone somatostatin, so milk stays in the stomach longer
- Boost insulin, which helps a baby use glucose, and gastrin, which releases stomach acid, boosts stomach movements and encourages gut lining cells to grow.

Another explanation is that a baby who practice-sucks spends more time being calm, which frees energy for growth.

PRACTICE-SUCKING FOR FORMULA-FED BABIES

If you're intending to bottle-feed, your baby can use a dummy for sucking practice.

FEEDING BY MOUTH

Your baby can start learning to drink by mouth if he's not on a ventilator, can co-ordinate breathing, swallowing and sucking, and has an efficient gag reflex.

Swallowing. A baby may be able to swallow after as little as 11 weeks in the womb!

Sucking. Some babies can suck as early as 18–24 weeks post-conception age. Jaundice and other health problems, or pethidine given in labour, sometimes temporarily dampen effective sucking. The older a baby's post-conception age, the more strongly he'll suck.

The gag reflex is a choke response which stops milk going down the wrong way and is present from 26–27 weeks post-conception age.

The rooting reflex is an instinctive lurching of a baby's mouth towards the breast, bottle or cup that appears in babies of more than 32 weeks post-conception age. If you stroke your baby's cheek near the corner of his mouth, then if he's alert and the rooting reflex is present, he'll turn towards your fingers and open his mouth wide like a baby bird gaping for a worm.

A baby who is old and mature enough to feed by mouth can feed from a cup, breast, breast plus nursing supplementer (see p. 73), or bottle.

As he grows he may use several methods, for example:

FOR A BREAST-MILK-FED BABY
- Cup alone
- Cup and breast. Ideally it's best to start cup and breast-feeding together
- Cup, breast and supplementer (see p. 73)
- Breast and supplementer
- Breast alone.

FOR A FORMULA-FED BABY
- Cup and bottle
- Bottle alone.

FOR A BABY FED BOTH BREAST MILK AND FORMULA
- Any of the above.

CUP-FEEDING (FROM 30–32 WEEKS)

In the past small babies were often fed with a spoon or dropper, but cup-feeding is better. Many prems can start at 30 weeks post-conception age, though some need to wait until 32 weeks.

Start teaching your baby to cup-feed with the feeding tube

in place, which means he may be tube- and cup-fed for several weeks. Babies like being cup-fed with breast milk because it's sweet.

IF YOU'RE SUPPLYING BREAST MILK

1 Shake the container of expressed breast milk and put some into a sterilised baby cup. Hold your baby on your lap – preferably by your naked breast so he smells you and your milk – and put a drop of milk on his tongue so he tastes its sweetness.
2 Gently tilt the cup so it touches the lower lip and a little milk enters his mouth – but take care not to swamp him. Within a few days or weeks he'll start lapping the milk like a kitten, or sipping or sucking it. Don't worry how much he takes; the nurses will work out whether he needs a top-up by tube.
3 Make this time as peaceful and relaxed as possible, so he associates cup-feeds with pleasure and tranquillity.

IF YOUR BABY IS FORMULA-FED

Do as above but with formula instead.

During the next few weeks your baby will take increasing amounts of milk from a cup and can start feeding from breast or bottle. He'll gradually need less and less by tube and the day will arrive when it can come out.

Some mothers never cup-feed but start teaching their babies to breastfeed with the tube in place (see p. 71).

Some units don't encourage cup-feeding.

BREASTFEEDING AND BOTTLE-FEEDING

Most babies need to weigh over 1500g (3lb 5oz) or be 32–34 weeks post-conception age to breastfeed or bottle-feed effectively, though some manage before. However, many babies start learning sooner than this.

If you want to bottle-feed, the nurses will advise you what sort of teat to use. As he becomes used to sucking milk from the bottle, and as he grows stronger, he'll take more and more at each feed until he can eventually stop cup-feeding.

BREAST MILK IN A BOTTLE RATHER THAN A CUP?

You or someone else could bottle-feed your baby with breast milk, but it isn't wise. A baby who learns to suck from a bottle may have difficulty adjusting to the different and more complex skills needed to suck and 'milk' the breast, and to adjust its flow.

HOW ABOUT ANOTHER MOTHER'S MILK? (see p. 67)

If your baby is very small, if you can't provide enough milk, even with skilled help, and if he isn't doing well on formula, then it's wise to give him donated breast milk – though it's an excellent idea to continue giving as much of your milk as you can.

Babies who particularly benefit from donated breast milk include:

- Very-low-birthweight tube-fed babies, especially in their first week, when they tolerate human milk better than formula
- Those not growing or thriving well
- Those who've had bowel surgery
- Those with a poorly functioning immune system, for example those who've already had an infection
- Those with diarrhoea
- Those with necrotising enterocolitis (see p. 99) – this is six to ten times more common in formula-fed babies, but donated milk is as protective as a mother's own milk.

Donated milk should ideally come from the mother of a baby of the same maturity as yours, so the composition of her milk is appropriate. However, such milk may be hard to find because most donated milk comes from mothers of full-term babies.

Donated milk is generally 'drip' milk – milk that drips from one breast while the mother is expressing or breastfeeding from the other. This is relatively low in fat and contains only two-thirds of the calories of expressed milk, so, ideally, a baby should have expressed milk.

DOES A BREASTFED BABY NEED FORMULA?

A breastfed baby doesn't need formula unless his mother can't provide enough milk. If your baby can't yet feed directly from the breast, you may find it difficult to produce enough. However, you can make more if you know how (see p. 66). And anyway, a little breast milk is always much better than none.

Your baby can have top-ups of pre-term formula unless there's a special reason for having donated milk. Babies fed breast milk and pre-term formula grow faster than those given breast milk and donated milk, possibly because donated milk is usually drip milk (see above), and because pasteurisation destroys the fat-releasing enzyme lipase (see p. 67).

WEIGHT GAIN

Don't worry when your baby loses weight after he's born. This weight loss is temporary and normal.

SUPPLEMENTS

The paediatrician may recommend supplements of vitamins (A, B, C, D, K and sometimes E and folic acid) for up to 6–12 months. A supplement of zinc is sometimes beneficial, too.

Now for some practical details of how to supply breast milk.

CHAPTER 7

Providing Breast Milk

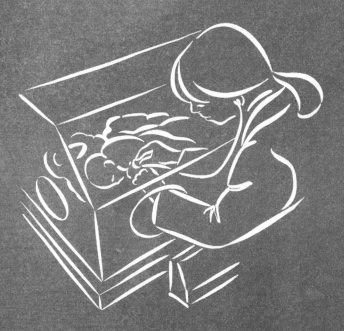

What makes you most likely to succeed at breastfeeding? The answer is *boosting and maintaining your milk supply by frequent expressing or pumping* – and doing this from very soon after she's born until she takes all she needs directly from the breast, which may be days, weeks or months.

Even then expressing (or, perhaps, pumping) can be very handy.

For the first one to four days after delivery you'll produce tiny amounts of colostrum – the early milk that's as valuable to your premature baby as liquid gold. It's worth reminding the nurses that you'd like her to receive your milk from the beginning, unless she's so immature or unwell that she needs intravenous feeds, in which case you should freeze your colostrum – yes, even just a few drops at a time – for later.

HOW TO EXPRESS YOUR MILK

Make sure you're in a warm room (no problem in the SCBU!), wash your hands, and encourage your milk to flow by relaxing, and by stroking your breasts and nipples. Being near your baby may help, or you could think about her or look at a photo of her.

Hold your areola with your thumb above and fingers below. Move your whole hand firmly back towards your chest. Now press your fingers and thumb together and move your hand away again, so as gently to squeeze out colostrum from the reservoirs under the areola.

When your milk 'comes in' (when your breasts start making the larger amounts of mature milk), these reservoirs may feel like tiny bunches of grapes, and a minute or so after you begin expressing you may notice your milk dripping or spraying out.

Move your hand round from time to time to empty all parts of the breast. If the flow slows, change to the other breast, and go from one to the other several times in a session so as to collect the richer milk from deep in the breast.

Catch the milk in a sterilised container. If left at room temperature, you should use it within six to eight hours; alternatively store it in the fridge for use within 24–48 hours, or in the freezer for use within three months. If you add a little milk to a container of frozen milk, cool the new milk first.

HOW OFTEN TO EXPRESS

In general, the more often you express, the more milk you'll make. Aim for every two to three hours during the day and arrange to do it at least eight times in each 24 hours. Never express less often than six times in 24 hours unless you want to reduce your supply. You may find you can sleep for six or seven hours without being woken by full breasts. This is fine if you can easily fit in eight expressions in 24 hours, but it's usually best at first to spread them out more and to express at least once at night.

the more often you express, the more milk you'll make

PUMPING MILK

It's best to express by hand for the first few days until your milk comes in. After that you can either continue with hand-expression or use a pump.

Get ready as described above for expressing – indeed you might like to encourage your milk to come by hand-expressing a bit first. You need to pump just as often as you'd hand-express. Many women pump for about ten minutes on each side – though some need more and others less. Switching from one breast to another every two or three minutes encourages the milk flow, but it's important to collect all the milk from each breast so your baby benefits from the deeper, richer milk.

Pumps are hand-operated or electric. Use whichever you find easier. If you're going to pump for some weeks, you may find an electric one more convenient. Some electric pumps allow you to pump both breasts at once.

HOW BREASTS MAKE MILK

The more often and the more effectively you empty your breasts, the more milk you'll make. Nipple stimulation during expression or pumping makes the brain's pituitary gland release a hormone called prolactin which instructs the breasts to make milk. The more time you spend expressing or pumping, the more prolactin and the more milk you'll make.

MAKING ENOUGH MILK

At first – and perhaps for the first few weeks – you'll make only small amounts. But you'll gradually produce more as you get into the swing of expressing or pumping. Don't worry if the amount varies – dwindling, for example, if you're worried about your baby. This is to be expected and you can increase your supply if you know how – ask the SCBU staff or a La Leche League leader or National Childbirth Trust breastfeeding counsellor, or read *Breast Is Best* (see p. 179).

You may well find you have some extra milk. You can donate this to a milk bank if your hospital has one.

Expressing or pumping in the early morning nearly always produces more milk than at other times. The 'lightest' times are generally in the evening.

If your baby needs more milk than you can express or pump, she can have a top-up with formula or donated breast milk.

BREAST-MILK BANKS

Donated breast milk is so valuable for some very small or unwell babies that it's sometimes transported from one hospital to another by road or rail.

A donor is carefully screened with blood tests for human immunodeficiency virus (HIV), hepatitis virus and other infections. And she's unsuitable if she's on drugs (including nicotine from smoking, alcohol, the Pill or aspirin).

Donated milk is checked to ensure that it has a sufficiently low bacteria count before being pasteurised and frozen for up to six months. Pasteurisation is best done by the 'flash' method. This helps protect antibodies and enzymes. However, pasteurisation destroys live cells, some vitamins and antibodies, and lipase – a fat-digesting enzyme which releases fatty acids. This lack of lipase means a baby drinking pasteurised donated milk grows more slowly than one fed raw (unpasteurised) milk. So, ideally, a needy small baby should have raw donated milk.

There's an address for information about milk banks on page 179.

EFFORT AND REWARD

Expressing and pumping are time-consuming and involve a lot of effort without the reward of having your baby at the breast. But hold on to the thought that you're giving her the very best start.

Hopefully, it won't be long before she starts breastfeeding.

Breastfeeding

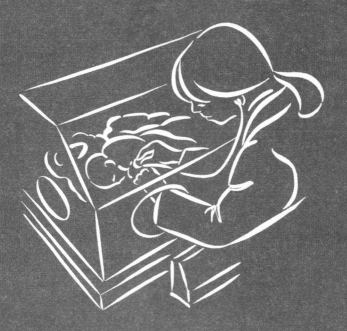

This chapter is for women whose low-birth-weight babies are sufficiently mature and well to start feeding directly from the breast.

This suggests a post-conception age of 30–35 weeks.

The earliest a baby can take milk directly from the breast is around 28 weeks (see p. 72), when he may lick drops of expressed milk from the nipple. By 30–32 weeks he may be able to swallow expressed, let-down or leaking milk that drips or flows while some of the areola is in his mouth. Eventually, perhaps between 32 and 34 weeks, he'll gradually start learning to suck and milk the breast himself.

You may like to find a relatively private, quiet corner in the SCBU or a mother's room nearby to help you relax while breastfeeding. Or you could use a screen or simply turn your chair away from other people if you wish. If you'd like a nurse with you, just ask. And if your baby is attached to a monitor and can't be disconnected while you feed, sit as near the monitor as possible.

There's information on familiarising your tube- and/or cup-fed baby with the breast in Chapter 6. This chapter outlines a few particularly important basics for breastfeeding a small baby.

EARLY SUCKLING (see p. 72)

If your newborn is mature and well enough to breastfeed, put him to the breast as soon as possible after birth. This allows both of you to take advantage of the strong sucking reflex present for 20–30 minutes immediately after birth. A strong sucking reflex should return after about 40 hours.

ENCOURAGING YOUR BABY TO BREAST-FEED

Knowing what to expect can make it easier to meet the challenge of getting enough milk into a small, immature baby.

For example, one who is mature enough to have a sucking reflex and well enough to start breastfeeding may:

- Be quickly tired by breastfeeding
- Feed better if you don't distract him by talking or stroking
- Be sleepy much of the time
- Fall asleep soon after starting a feed
- Refuse to carry on feeding before the milk has started to flow
- Refuse to carry on feeding when the milk starts to flow
- Not make his hunger known (for example, by restlessness or crying – what some call 'demanding' a feed) until 40 weeks post-conception.

'ISLANDS OF WAKEFULNESS'

It's clearly easier to breastfeed if you're with your baby as much as possible, so you can put him to the breast in the short periods of time when he's awake and alert. It's often best to catch his natural 'islands of wakefulness' when you can, rather than wake him artificially for a feed, because he'll grow better if he sleeps a lot. However, if your baby doesn't wake often enough, you will need to wake him gently.

BREASTFEEDING A BABY WHO'S STILL CUP-FED AND/OR TUBE-FED

Wash your hands before putting your baby to the breast, wrap him up if you like, make yourself comfy, and hold him so he's facing your chest without twisting his neck. The nurses can help you position him so your breast doesn't get in the way of his nose, so he doesn't drag on the nipple, and so he can take the breast ('latch on') if and when he wants.

AT 28 WEEKS POST-CONCEPTION

Try putting him to the breast perhaps a couple of times a day to see if he's interested in licking drops of milk expressed from the nipple. He can have a tube-feed at the same time (see p. 56). If your breast is full or hard, express a little milk first to take the pressure off, otherwise the flow might make him choke. Softening the breast also means that some of the areola will fit in his mouth if he sucks.

Remember, he can't breastfeed yet. All he'll do is practise being at the breast, learn to enjoy being there, taste the milk and perhaps hold the nipple and areola in his mouth. If he sucks at all, he'll probably do little bursts of three to five rapid, practice, 'non-nutritive' sucks which don't draw any milk out. After several sporadic bursts of this he'll stop, tired out.

AT 30–32 WEEKS POST-CONCEPTION

As above, but also try expressing a few drops of milk directly into his mouth before or during a tube-feed or before a cup-feed.

AT 32–34 WEEKS POST-CONCEPTION

When he shows an interest, encourage him to open his mouth wide and take the breast further in. He'll still do plenty of practice sucks, but at some stage he'll gradually start learning to breastfeed effectively by sucking and by 'milking' – removing milk from the reservoirs beneath the areola by massaging the breast with his tongue and jaw. As he grows older and stronger, he'll get more used to breastfeeding and more able to co-ordinate breathing, sucking and swallowing, so he'll gradually take more and more milk. However, learning to breastfeed effectively usually takes babies this immature many weeks.

A few babies this age occasionally take one or more full

feeds from the breast in 24 hours – each of the same amount they would have had in a tube-feed. It's still very early days, but knowing your baby is getting what he needs from a cup and, possibly, a tube as well means there's no pressure on you or him to perform. So don't let anyone put you off. There's no competition and no reason why your baby should be brilliant at breastfeeding when by rights he shouldn't even

> *There's no competition and no reason why your baby should be brilliant at breastfeeding when by rights he shouldn't even be born yet!*

be born yet! Many full-term babies take several months to become effective breastfeeders, and yours needs to catch up on the time he missed in the womb.

AT 35–37 WEEKS POST-CONCEPTION

Eventually, your baby will take so much milk from the breast that you can discard the cup and/or tube.

USING A SUPPLEMENTER

Some mothers find that using a gadget called a supplementer – also known as a 'nursing' (breastfeeding) supplementer – helps their tube-fed baby learn to breastfeed and makes using a cup unnecessary.

A supplementer (see p. 180) consists of a small polythene bag – which you fill with breast milk and pin on your clothing high above the breast – with two fine tubes of a size chosen to produce the required milk flow coming from the bag and going one to each nipple. Each tube is taped to the breast so one end protrudes very slightly beyond the nipple and enters the baby's mouth when he breastfeeds.

Although the baby isn't mature or strong enough to get all the milk he needs directly from the breast, taking breast milk from the supplementer at the same time means he becomes used to the idea of filling his tummy at the breast. And at the same time he stimulates your breasts – and therefore your milk supply.

As he becomes stronger, bigger and more mature, he'll gradually suck and 'milk' your breasts more efficiently until the naso-gastric tube can eventually go, and one day the supplementer, too.

DIFFERENT POSITIONS

Once you're confident with feeding in one position, it's a good idea to get used to feeding in different positions. This helps prevent any one part of the breast being emptied better than any other, and also helps prevent nipple soreness and cracks.

For example, experiment with:

- The 'football' (or underarm) hold – with his legs under your arm on the side you're feeding
- Him sitting upright on a pile of cushions on your lap and facing your breast
- You both lying down, with him either the same side as the breast you're feeding from, or the other side, with you leaning over.

HOW OFTEN?

If your baby is mature and strong enough to take all his feeds directly from the breast, use his 'islands of wakefulness' to fit in *at least* eight feeds in 24 hours, and as many more as he wants. Many feed ten times in 24 hours and some as often as 14 times a day, though with napping and practice-sucking it's hard to tell when a 'feed' is over. Babies need particularly frequent feeds when they have a growth spurt.

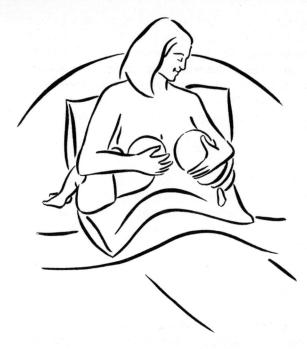

If you can't manage even eight feeds, make up the difference with sessions of expressing or pumping. The more often you feed, the more milk you'll make and the quicker your baby will become good at breastfeeding – as long as he gets enough sleep and doesn't get overtired.

Night feeds of breast milk are important to your baby, and for you – to encourage your milk supply. If you don't want to wake more than once, the staff can cup-feed the baby with your expressed or pumped milk.

ONE BREAST OR TWO?

A premature baby gets tired so quickly that he'll probably manage to feed from only one breast at a time. When he's older he'll be able to go to the second breast and may switch from one to the other several times. Sometimes, though, he may be perfectly satisfied with one.

If your baby has a very short feed and then drops off to sleep, express or pump the rest of the milk from that breast. Put it into a named, dated container labelled 'rich milk'. Then express or pump all the milk from the other breast into another named and dated container. (However, if you're making too much milk, don't express or pump the other breast, but simply start that side at the next feed.)

Store the containers of milk safely, as directed by the nurses, and the next time he wakes give him the saved 'rich' milk first, by tube, cup or supplementer. This allows him to get the fattier, higher-calorie milk he needs to grow. A baby who has repeated short feeds gets only the relatively watery, low-calorie early milk which contains a lot of lactose (milk sugar). He won't grow as well as he could and might have colic and diarrhoea because of its high lactose content.

HOW TO TELL WHEN HE'S HAD ENOUGH

It can be difficult to know when a learner breastfeeder has had enough because:

- He's too young as yet to breastfeed for long and may keep dropping off and waking again. This doesn't matter if you have the time and patience. If you get bored, you may find it helps to watch TV
- Much (or all, in a very immature baby) of his sucking is non-nutritive, practice sucking
- The rate of milk flow can vary from 1ml (a fifth of a level teaspoonful – just a few drops) a minute to as much as 13ml (nearly a tablespoonful) a minute in some women when letting their milk down.

Some experts recommend weighing a low-birthweight learner

breastfeeder before and after a feed so as to work out how much milk he's taken; if he hasn't had enough, he can then have a top-up of expressed milk by tube or cup. Don't worry if your baby doesn't take much directly from you. You can increase your milk supply by expressing or pumping more. And he'll learn to take more as he grows stronger and more mature.

NIPPLE CARE

Look after your nipples by:
- Making sure your baby is well positioned and takes as much of the areola into his mouth as possible
- Changing his position from feed to feed
- Giving frequent feeds (yes, *frequent* – research shows that nipples toughen up faster with frequent feeds than with infrequent ones)
- Keeping your nipples as dry as you can between feeds by exposing them to the air or changing your breast pads frequently
- Not using soap on them.

LEAKING

Many breastfeeding mothers of prems produce more milk than their baby needs and find themselves leaking or letting down unexpectedly when their breasts are full.
　You can deal with this by:
- Expressing or pumping just enough milk to take the pressure off – but not too much, as this stimulates even greater milk production
- Using breast pads
- Putting a plastic breast shell (available from the nurses or, if not, by order from a pharmacy) inside your bra to collect leaking milk. You can store this for use by your baby or by

someone else's, but remember that it's 'early' milk and not as rich as that produced later in a feed.

ENGORGEMENT

In the early days of producing milk your breasts may become swollen, tense and tender. Prevent this by expressing or pumping just enough to take the pressure off as soon as you notice them becoming at all uncomfortable.

GETTING HELP

Some babies have particular problems which affect their ability to breastfeed, and their mothers may need special help as they learn to meet the challenge. Having twins may mean you need skilled help to sort out the practicalities of breastfeeding, too.

But most breastfeeding women experience challenges of one sort or another. Among the most frequent are sore nipples and a blocked duct. It pays to have ready access to information. You can get this from nurses and midwives skilled at breastfeeding help, or from a breastfeeding helper trained by the National Childbirth Trust or La Leche League (see pp. 177, 178). There's detailed information about breastfeeding in *Breast Is Best* and *Breastfeeding Special Care Babies* (see p. 179).

Now to 'kangaroo-care' – a special way of looking after babies that encourages them to breastfeed and is rewarding for bottle-feeders, too.

CHAPTER 9

Kangaroo-care

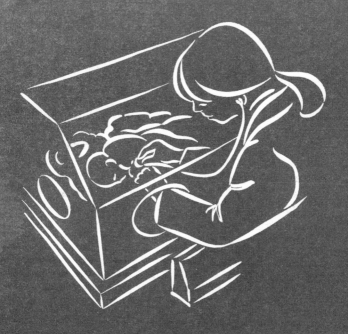

Some low-birthweight babies benefit from being nursed next to their mother's skin, inside her clothes.

Like baby kangaroos, these newborns enjoy the warmth and physical closeness of their mothers; they also sleep better and have fewer illnesses. And it can be very pleasant to have such intimate contact with your baby.

WHERE IT ORIGINATED

Kangaroo-care isn't new. Around the world mothers have cuddled their babies close and wrapped them inside their clothes since time immemorial, especially if the babies are small, frail or unwell. What *is* new is that many paediatricians and nurses now encourage kangaroo-care for small babies.

many paediatricians and nurses now encourage kangaroo-care for small babies

The trend began in Bogota, Colombia, where two paediatricians were alarmed by so many babies dying. Their hospital couldn't afford enough incubators, and putting several babies together encouraged cross-infection. So they used the facilities already on hand – the mothers themselves – because kangaroo-care provides an incubator-like environment but with the added benefit of the mother's presence and vigilance.

30 POSSIBLE BENEFITS OF KANGAROO-CARE

Studies show that a kangaroo-care baby may:
1 Be healthier
2 Grow better
3 Leave her incubator earlier
4 Leave the SCBU a little sooner
5 Go home sooner
6 Maintain a steadier temperature
7 Benefit from breathing the humid air inside her mother's clothing
8 Have a reduced risk of 'stop-breathing' (apnoea) attacks
9 Have less risk of an oxygen shortage
10 Relax more because of her mother's smell, feel, sounds and movement
11 Enjoy it so much that a look of blissful contentment and peace comes over her as she snuggles in
12 Be less restless and use less energy
13 Sleep more deeply
14 Cry less now and six months later
15 Search for the breast earlier
16 Be more interested in breastfeeding
17 Boost – perhaps even double – her mother's milk production
18 Interest her mother in expressing milk for weeks longer
19 Encourage her mother not to stop breastfeeding
20 Have a smaller risk of regurgitating and inhaling milk
21 Allow her mother to be more closely involved
22 Have more 'islands of wakefulness'
23 Have more chance of a feed when most ready for one
24 Have her needs met quicker because of her mother's constant vigilance
25 Give and receive more eye-contact
26 Have less risk of a slow heartbeat (bradycardia)

27 Be protected from bright light by her mother's clothes
28 Be protected from infection – because fewer people
    touch her, she's more likely to receive breast milk, and her
    relaxed state strengthens her immune system
29 Have a greater chance of surviving if in a developing
    country
30 Save the hospital money.

HOW BIG MUST SHE BE?

In developing countries some babies as light as 500g (1lb 2oz)
benefit from kangaroo-care. In the UK, it's generally encouraged or allowed only if a baby is at least 27 weeks post-
conception age and weighs over 1000g (2lb 3oz).

But for a very small or unwell baby it isn't a substitute for
intensive care.

WHAT ABOUT TUBES AND WIRES?

Kangaroo-care for some of the day is suitable for many babies
in incubators, even if they have tubes and wires attached, and
require tube-feeding or extra oxygen – even CPAP (see p. 21).
The only proviso is that the mother must sit near the equipment to which her baby is attached.

If it's safe for the staff to detach your baby from the tubes
and wires, you can walk around with her, too.

WHAT TO WEAR

You wear normal clothes, with a shirt or jumper but no bra as
it's best for your baby to nestle against your bare chest. She
wears just a nappy and hat.

HOW TO POSITION HER

Put her chest and tummy against your chest, between your breasts, with her head perhaps turned to one side, and snuggle her close with your arms around her. If you're sitting down, put a blanket around her, over your clothes, and hold her in place.

HOW TO MAKE HER SECURE

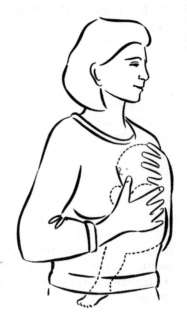

If you want your arms free, or want to walk around, the nurses will help you secure her to your chest so she can't fall out.

One way is to fold a square piece of cloth (such as a piece of a sheet) into a triangle, then to tie the long side around you and the baby, and to tuck the bottom point up and under her. You can hold her bottom for added security.

Another way is to put her inside your jumper and put a belt round your waist.

WHEN TO PUT HER IN AN INCUBATOR OR COT

If the staff agree, you can keep her in the kangaroo position as long as you like, removing her only to change her nappy, or to put her back in the incubator or cot when you need a break or the staff need to attend to her.

Alternatively, the nurses may recommend kangaroo-care for perhaps half an hour to one hour at a time, once or twice a day.

WHAT ABOUT FEEDING?

A tube-fed or cup-fed baby can have feeds right where she is – in her 'pouch'.

As for breastfeeding, you may find you can feed your baby simply by moving her slightly. The ease of breastfeeding is one reason why kangaroo-care is often so successful.

WHAT ABOUT TWINS?

Kangaroo-care is ideal for twins.

CAN ANYONE ELSE DO IT?

Your partner or a nurse can also provide kangaroo-care. This is better for many babies than being isolated in an incubator or cot and produces many of the benefits mentioned above. A nurse wouldn't put your baby next to her bare skin but would secure her with a sheet over her clothing.

> *Your partner or a nurse can also provide kanga-roo-care.*

Now to the practicalities of everyday life with your baby in hospital.

CHAPTER 10

Daily Life

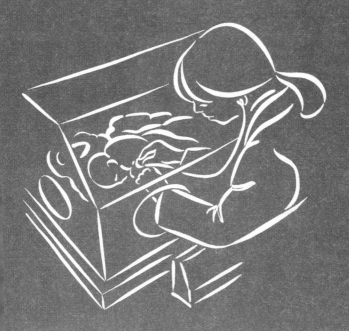

Having a premature baby transforms you into being a newborn's parent prematurely. This may be a challenge, for unlike parents of full-terms, many parents of prems must cope with the SCBU.

On the positive side, they know their baby is getting good care and have ongoing backup as they adjust to unexpectedly early parenthood.

LIVING IN HOSPITAL

It's easier to spend time in the SCBU if you stay in hospital. This also makes it easier to supply breast milk and to breast-feed, and enables you to be there for night-time feeds. It's especially helpful if your baby is in a hospital some distance from your home.

The hospital may become your temporary home for some days, weeks or, for a few mothers, months, so you'll need to find ways of making eating, bathing, phoning and relaxing as easy and pleasant as possible. The nurses and other mothers will give you tips and, if you aren't happy with anything, you can ask a hospital manager if matters can be improved. You can come and go from hospital as you wish. And if you have your own room, your partner may be able to stay, too, though you'll be squashed in a single bed!

Some mothers with a baby in the SCBU become so used to institutionalised life that they forget what it's like to be an independent person capable of choices and decisions. This can create problems for partners who expect them to be the same as before. Being aware of this possible friction can help keep your relationship on an even keel.

HOME ALONE

You may not stay in hospital because there's no room, or you have other demands on your time. Some women feel isolated at home without their baby, especially if it's their first, and you may want company. You can phone the special care unit when you want, and it's a good idea to give the staff your number – or a contact number – so you don't feel cut off.

Carry on expressing or pumping milk – borrowing, hiring or buying a pump if necessary – ask the SCBU staff for details. You can take or send milk to your baby each day, or freeze it and take or send it when you can. Providing milk helps you feel involved and means you know you're doing the best for him. Don't forget to label the container with the date, time and baby's name.

If you're close enough to visit your baby frequently, take special care of yourself (see Chapter 5). Splitting your time between home and hospital and travelling between the two makes this a busy, challenging time, and you'll cope best if you don't expect to be a superwoman but are kind to yourself and ask for any help you need.

Not everyone can visit their baby frequently or stay long while there. They may live too far away; the journey on public transport may be too difficult; they may not have fully recovered from pregnancy and labour; or they may have other responsibilities, such as young children. It can be frustrating to be apart from your baby so much, but if you phone the staff each day they'll keep you informed. When your baby eventually comes home, you'll get to know each other more intimately and form a good bond.

Your body needs time to restore itself after childbirth. Many mothers find it takes a long time – a year is not uncommon –

to adjust and feel as full of energy as before pregnancy. And with the challenges of caring for a premature baby it may take even longer.

HOLDING, ENJOYING AND CARING FOR HIM

Most parents find the biggest rewards of having a baby are the simple pleasures that come from holding, cuddling, feeding and caring for him – and enjoying those first direct gazes and, later, smiles.

PATERNITY LEAVE

In the UK three months of statutory unpaid paternity leave will be enforced by the year 2000. If your partner can't arrange time off and you have other children, you'll have to go home if you're well enough. And if you have to stay in hospital, you'll need someone else to care for them. Relatives and neighbours are the best bet, but Social Services can arrange temporary foster care.

Some fathers become very involved with their baby's care and progress. They visit frequently, share care and hold their baby kangaroo-style.

Others find that becoming a father of a baby needing special care is disruptive and stressful, and need 'special care' and consideration themselves.

YOUR OTHER CHILDREN

If you stay in hospital and have other children, try to go home to see them as often as possible, or have someone bring them in most days, if not every day. The early arrival of their new brother or sister may be thrilling but it is also a surprise, if not a shock, and they may have mixed feelings.

They'll adjust more easily to your absence and preoccupation with the baby if you involve them. And they'll need someone to listen and give them attention if they're not to become jealous.

It'll help if they know what to expect of the baby when he comes home. Many children are disappointed to find it's a long time before a full-term baby walks and talks, let alone runs around and plays football! And they'll have to wait even longer before a prem catches up.

Ideas to help young children adjust include:

- Buying a doll for them to look after like a premature baby – perhaps with a home-made cardboard box incubator
- Reading *Special Care Babies* (see p. 179)
- Giving the baby one of their toys
- Making a tape of them talking to the baby
- Filling in a chart with details of the baby's growth
- Play-acting how much the baby will do when he comes home

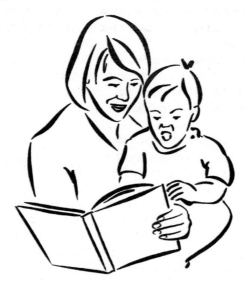

- Remembering what they've learnt since *they* were born
- Making a scrapbook or storyboard about the baby
- Drawing a nameplate for the incubator
- Doing pictures for the inside of the incubator
- Choosing an outfit for the baby
- Enjoying outings and activities which have nothing to do with babies!

WHAT ABOUT WORK?

Some people claim that most women with babies want to work. But a careful look at what women choose to do when offered the opportunity of work and child-care shows this isn't true. *Most women want to be with their babies.*

However, those who want to work, or want to work when their children are older – which increasing numbers do – want arrangements as mother-and-child-friendly as possible. They may choose to work:

- Part-time
- At home
- Near home – with very little commuting
- Where they can take their child
- Somewhere with a good nursery
- Only if a trusted and known person – such as a relative or friend – cares for their child.

But work is the last thing on the minds of most mothers of babies in special care, and some need all their energy to face challenges to their babies' health and well-being.

CHAPTER 11

Early Challenges

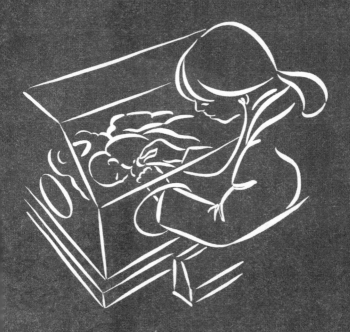

The vast majority of low-birthweight babies do very well. However, the smaller and less mature a baby is, the more likely she is to encounter certain challenges or complications. And each reacts to these in her own unique way.

BREATHING PROBLEMS

Around one premature baby in ten has a breathing problem, and the earlier she's born, the more likely this is.

Possible reasons include:
- Small, immature lungs
- Weak breathing muscles
- A soft ribcage
- 'Stop-breathing' (apnoea) attacks (see p. 19)
- The respiratory distress syndrome
- A hole in the membrane around a lung, making it collapse (pneumothorax)
- Brain damage
- Pneumonia.

Untreated breathing problems lead to a shortage of oxygen (hypoxia) which, if prolonged, severe or untreated, can damage various parts of the body such as the eyes, ears or brain. SCBU staff watch for hypoxia by monitoring a baby's breathing and heart rate and measuring blood gas levels (see pp. 20 and 23). They also help prevent or correct it with extra oxygen, CPAP and, if necessary, ventilation (see p. 21).

RESPIRATORY DISTRESS SYNDROME (RDS)

This develops in four out of five babies born before 30 weeks, generally within the first four hours of life, and overall it affects about 12,000 babies a year in the UK. Delaying premature labour so a mother can receive steroids (see p. 8) reduces the risk, possibly by stimulating the baby's production of surfactant (see below).

Researchers are also investigating whether giving a pre-term baby steroids lowers the risk of chronic lung disease (see below).

Surfactant: A baby's lungs begin to make surfactant from 22 weeks of pregnancy, and at 34–36 weeks there's a big rise in production. This fatty substance is a lubricant which lowers the surface tension of the moisture lining the airways. This keeps the tiny air spaces open and helps a baby breathe.

But a baby born before 36 weeks may not make enough for a few days after birth. This leads to the rapid, grunting breathing characteristic of RDS. Three in four babies with RDS need ventilation.

Surfactant may also be lacking if an unborn baby 'poohs' meconium (early bowel contents) into the amniotic fluid. This fluid fills her lungs, but any meconium inactivates surfactant.

Doctors can now put artificial surfactant into a baby's lungs to help prevent or treat RDS. Without treatment, one in four babies born before 28 weeks dies within a month, and one in four develops chronic lung disease.

CHRONIC LUNG DISEASE

Lung damage reduces gas exchange, strains the heart and means help with breathing is essential. If a baby needs oxygen for more than 28 days, or still needs it at the time she would have been 36 weeks if still in the womb, she is said to have chronic lung disease (broncho-pulmonary dysplasia, BPD).

This is more likely in babies:

- Born before 28 weeks
- On a ventilator a long time – because of the high air pressures necessary to inflate the lungs
- Needing a high oxygen concentration
- Needing high-pressure ventilation.

Most babies need less extra oxygen as their lungs heal, though some still need it when they go home – and a few for up to two years.

BRAIN DAMAGE

An unborn baby's brain size quadruples between 24 and 40 weeks. The brain of a premature baby – especially one born before 28 weeks – is smaller, less well developed and more vulnerable than that of a full-term baby.

During an oxygen shortage brain cells are protected to some extent by getting a bigger share of the body's blood flow.

Mild brain damage often goes unnoticed. However, more serious and permanent damage is a particular hazard for very small babies. Some types of brain damage are similar to that suffered by adults during a stroke. Others cause more widespread problems. At worst a baby may have one or more of several disabilities, including defective eyesight, cerebral palsy and, later in childhood perhaps, clumsiness (dyspraxia), a poor attention span (attention deficit disorder), speech problems and learning difficulties.

Brain damage has several possible causes:

Lack of oxygen (hypoxia). The smaller a baby is, the more likely a lack of oxygen is to damage the brain.

Before and during birth, several problems can reduce a baby's oxygen supply by slowing the placental blood flow to the two arteries in the umbilical cord. For example:

- An unhealthy placenta (see p. 132)
- Premature separation of the placenta (abruption) interrupts the placental blood vessels
- A squashed umbilical cord (for example, during a breech birth or an overlong delivery).

A lack of oxygen during labour alone accounts for only a small proportion of the number of babies with brain damage.

After birth, several other problems can arise, including:

- Breathing difficulties
- Prolonged 'stop-breathing' (apneoa) attacks
- Slowing of the heart rate.

Bleeding into the brain or its fluid-filled spaces. This may result from:

- Physical forces during a difficult birth tearing delicate blood vessels
- A lack of oxygen (see above)
- High or low blood pressure in the baby.

Bleeding in the first week is relatively common in babies born before 33 weeks, occurring in one in four born before 25 weeks. It tends to be worse in very premature babies because their blood doesn't clot as it should. But the good news is that even an extensive bleed sometimes leaves no permanent damage, and many lesser bleeds cause no noticeable problems.

A *feverish illness in the mother during pregnancy*. Researchers have uncovered a link between a high fever, and brain damage in an unborn baby.

Iodine deficiency. If a pregnant woman has an iodine-deficient diet, this can affect her baby's brain development and permanently reduce the potential to learn. Such a diet is rare in the UK nowadays.

A *low thyroid hormone level before or after birth*. Routine blood tests after birth can detect a low thyroid hormone level. This can then be treated.

Low blood sugar (see p. 23).

Jaundice (see p. 100).

NEW RESEARCH INTO BRAIN DAMAGE

- If blood gas tests reveal a shortage of oxygen, researchers can detect whether the brain is also short of oxygen, or not working properly, by shining infra-red light through the baby's head (see also p. 11). Red, oxygen-rich blood in the head absorbs a different amount of this light compared with blue, oxygen-poor blood. Computer analysis of the emerging light pattern indicates any oxygen-starved parts of the brain; a similar technique indicates which parts of the brain respond to stimulation.

- If a brain scan indicates potential damage from a shortage of oxygen, researchers hope that starting to cool the baby's head within the first six hours will reduce the brain's need for oxygen until the crisis is over, and help prevent brain cell death. They say this is a possibility because permanent brain damage does not occur immediately after a shortage of oxygen, but takes up to 48 hours to develop. Cooling also prevents oxygen-starved cells continuing (perhaps for weeks) to release damaging chemicals. Wearing a 'cooling cap' for 12–72 hours safely cools a baby's head by 3–4°C, to around 32°C. (The rest of her body must be warmed to prevent hypothermia.) Researchers believe the

permanent brain damage does not occur immediately after a shortage of oxygen

danger is over after 24 hours and that the oxygen-starved cells can then heal.

CEREBRAL PALSY

Very-low-birthweight babies are the most likely to develop brain damage leading to cerebral palsy, and an ultrasound or MRI (magnetic resonance imaging) scan can identify those most at risk. The severity and signs of cerebral palsy vary but it usually shows up as stiffness, involuntary movements, or poor co-ordination and balance.

One in four babies with cerebral palsy has had a severe lack of oxygen during birth; some develop epilepsy and mental retardation, too. Another cause is a pre-existing problem (for example, a malformation) which affects movement and muscle tension in the womb, encourages a baby to settle into the breech position and leads to an oxygen shortage from a difficult birth.

BLEEDING PROBLEMS

Many premature babies bleed easily because:
- They may have **too few platelets** (tiny blood particles which aid clotting) particularly if they have an infection or their mother has severe pre-eclampsia
- Their delicate blood vessels bleed more easily from mechanical stresses during a difficult birth
- Their delicate blood vessels bleed more easily if an oxygen lack leads to a compensatory increase in the brain's blood flow.

ANAEMIA

Premature babies have no iron stores and easily become anaemic, especially if their mother bled from the placenta before labour, there's a rhesus problem or very frequent blood samples are taken. However, transfusions of carefully screened blood can put this right.

RETINOPATHY OF PREMATURITY

Some prems weighing less than 1000g (2lb 3oz) develop an eye condition called retinopathy of prematurity (ROP), previously known as retrolental fibroplasia. These babies are so immature that the tiny blood vessels at the back of their eyes haven't yet grown – like a spider's web – from the centre of the retina to its outskirts.

When such a baby starts receiving higher levels of oxygen (either from air or from extra oxygen) than are normal in the womb, the outer, bare areas of each retina produce chemicals which stimulate the blood vessels to grow in the wrong direction – into the jelly which fills the eye instead of into the outer, bare areas of retina.

As blood vessels grow into the jelly they may bleed and create scars which impair vision. These scars may also pull the retina away from the back of the eye, and without treatment this can, at worst, make the baby blind.

One baby in two weighing less than 1000g (2lb 3oz) may get ROP, as do most born before 26 weeks. The good news is that nine out of ten recover, though a few need laser treatment of their retina ten weeks later.

One baby in two weighing less than 1000g (2lb 3oz) may get ROP

The signs of ROP are visible to a doctor who examines the retina with an ophthalmoscope. They first show six or seven weeks after birth and reach their height by ten weeks. In some hospitals all babies born before 31 weeks and/or weighing less than 1500g are screened every two weeks from about seven weeks after birth until they reach 36 weeks post-conception age.

Possible causes of ROP include:
- Breathing a high concentration of oxygen (no longer used for small babies)
- Very low birthweight.

Researchers are also examining the idea that very intense lighting in SCBUs (see p. 36) may damage a baby's eyes by creating in the retina unstable particles called free radicals.

INFECTIONS

Premature babies are much more likely to develop infections (for example, pneumonia and gastroenteritis) because their immune systems are relatively immature. Breastfeeding reduces this risk.

NECROTISING ENTEROCOLITIS (NEC)

This inflammation and destruction of the bowel lining is associated with a reduced blood flow and infection in the bowel. Sadly, it kills one or two in every five affected babies.

Several factors make it more likely, including:
- Shortage of oxygen before birth (for example, with severe pre-eclampsia and an altered blood flow in the umbilical cord). This reduces the bowel's blood supply (because the body directs blood to the brain to protect it)
- Prematurity
- Low birthweight – four out of five babies with NEC weigh under 2500g (5lb 8oz), and up to 13 per cent of very-low-birthweight babies are affected
- Formula-feeding
- Frequent 'stop-breathing' attacks
- Frequent slowing of the heartbeat
- Frequent infections
- Persistent ductus arteriosus (see below).

Staff carefully watch babies with any of these factors for the many possible signs of NEC. Treatment is with intravenous fluids or feeds, and antibiotics. Very few babies require surgery.

JAUNDICE

Four out of five premature babies develop jaundice (yellowing of skin and eyes), compared with one in two full-terms. By far the commonest cause is 'physiological' jaundice. This often happens in the first few days because the immature liver allows a yellow pigment, bilirubin, to accumulate in the blood. This is usually harmless and the jaundice gradually disappears. However, a very high level can, at worst, damage the brain, so doctors treat it with blue light (see p. 22) until it falls, usually after three to ten days. In the rare event that it remains very high, an exchange transfusion may be necessary.

Jaundice persisting for two weeks or more needs further investigation as it may have another cause, such as liver or thyroid disease.

HEART FAILURE

In some of the smallest babies the stress of being alive causes heart failure.

CONGENITAL DISORDERS

Premature babies have a higher risk of several congenital disorders (developmental abnormalities present at birth). One such is patent ductus arteriosus (PDA), in which the blood vessel (ductus arteriosus) connecting the body's main artery (aorta) with the artery carrying blood from the heart to the lungs (pulmonary artery) stays open after birth. This either prevents blood going to the lungs to collect oxygen and release carbon dioxide, or, if blood flows the other way, may allow too much blood to go to the lungs.

At worst – and especially in very premature babies – PDA leads to problems such as heart failure and necrotising enterocolitis. Treatment may involve giving extra oxygen until the PDA closes, or giving a drug such as indomethacin which narrows it. More than three in five babies born before 25 weeks need drug treatment. A few need surgery.

DECIDING WHETHER TO TREAT YOUR BABY ANY MORE

In spite of the very best of medical attention and nursing care, a few babies deteriorate and become very unwell. It may then become clear that a baby is dying, or that further treatment may just keep her alive but at too great a cost to her long-term health.

If this happens to you and your baby, the doctors and yourselves as parents may have to make some difficult decisions about whether to continue or initiate treatment. The medical staff will do their best to keep you constantly involved in the decision-making and informed about your baby's condition.

This can be an almost unbearably emotional time. You'll probably feel helpless in the face of the impending tragedy. And even knowing that everyone did all they

You can choose who is present to support you and your partner

could may seem scant comfort, because living through a child's dying and death is one of the worst things to happen to a parent.

You may want to help the doctors plan when to withdraw treatment – for example, when to turn off the ventilator.

You can choose who is present to support you and your partner and to join in the farewell – perhaps a relative, a favourite nurse or doctor, the hospital chaplain, your other children or a friend. You may want special lighting, a reading, a song or other music, prayers or something else to help you with your parting.

You can cuddle your baby as she dies and for as long as you want afterwards. And you may even find your experience a time of grace and special blessing.

The staff in some SCBUs make it possible for parents to return the next day to see and cuddle their dead baby one last time. (See also page 109).

Now on to how parents of premature and small-for-dates babies can best deal with their reactions.

CHAPTER 12

Managing Your Reactions

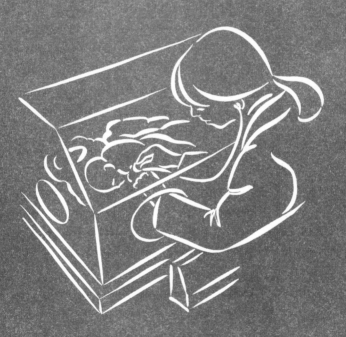

Having a baby produces a whole range of emotions, but having one prematurely can be even more emotional.

How you and your partner react will depend on many things, including your personalities, hopes and expectations, experience of birth and bereavement, professional and social support, and relationships with each other and with family, friends and staff.

RECOGNISING HOW YOU FEEL

Many people find that recognising their emotions helps them pull through, so try ticking any of the following states that ring bells for you:
• Surprised
• Excited
• Delighted
• Happy
• Hopeful
• Proud
• Thrilled
• Awestruck
• 'Slayed' by joy
• Protective
• Overwhelmed
• Distressed
• Unprepared
• Helpless
• Powerless
• Out of control
• Different from other parents

- Inadequate – can't cope
- Incapable – don't know what to do
- Inferior – other people are better at this than me
- Insecure
- Intimidated – by the environment of the SBCU
- Frustrated
- Isolated, lost or alone
- Daunted
- Stunned or dazed – with no feelings for some days, weeks or even months
- Shocked
- Confused
- Disappointed
- Alarmed
- Stressed
- Underconfident
- A failure
- Angry – at not having a 'normal' baby; some parents project this anger on to someone else
- Jealous – of the nurses caring for your baby
- Guilty – because part of you didn't want the baby, or you think you contributed to your baby's prematurity
- Perplexed – as you search for a cause
- Resentful – 'Why me?'
- Yearning – for the 'normal' baby you expected
- Anxious
- Apprehensive – about the unknown
- Frightened – that your baby may die or be permanently unwell or disabled
- Sad – about your baby's predicament
- Despairing
- Regretful – at losing the life you once had
- Cheated – of the last bit of pregnancy
- Unmotherly
- Detached.

The good news about a maelstrom of emotions is that it will subside in time as you come to terms with what's happened.

HOW YOUR BABY LOOKS

Some women immediately fall for their babies, but others feel little and a few are even repulsed. For the more premature a baby is, the more different he looks from a full-term one. Prems should, by rights, still be in the womb, and a baby younger than 30 weeks can look scrawny, skinny and positively 'fetal'. A tiny baby is fascinating and amazing but not necessarily appealing and somehow looks old before his time.

A tiny baby is fascinating and amazing but not necessarily appealing and somehow looks old before his time.

His eyes may bulge, dart around and be closed a lot; his face is bony rather than sweetly plump, and his ears may easily be pressed out of shape. The eyelids may (at 24–25 weeks) still be joined and the brows and lashes absent. His skin may be transparent and wrinkled, with visible blood vessels, and may look red, pale, grey or bluish; he may have dark downy hair (lanugo) all over, including his face, until 37–38 weeks post-conception age. Toenails don't start appearing until 32–36 weeks. Any breathing problems make him grunt and breathe rapidly, with a heaving chest, flared nostrils and flesh sucked in between his ribs. He may yawn or hiccup a lot. And he may temporarily have splayed-out arms and legs, small genitals, a small chest and a big tummy.

The good news is that he'll look better and better as the weeks pass.

COMMUNICATION

Good communication, with careful listening, clear statements about your needs or wants, and encouragement, will enhance your relationships with your partner, children and SCBU staff.

Effective listening has three important stages:

1 Listen to yourself and name *your* feelings. Then if you wish, put them to one side while you focus on listening to someone else
2 Try to be aware of and to name their feelings
3 Pass your hunch by them. If wrong, they'll put you right and be pleased you care enough to try to fathom how they're feeling.

ENCOURAGEMENT AND SUPPORT

If possible, encourage the staff, your partner, children and visitors by commenting on what's good about what they do for you and your baby. And accept any encouragement you receive with good grace!

You may find that you and other SCBU parents form a support group, listening, encouraging and perhaps having a laugh over a coffee or something stronger.

LAUGHTER

It's surprising where humour can be found. And you'll be delighted by the difference it sometimes makes.

POSTNATAL DEPRESSION

Many women feel low with 'baby blues' for up to ten days after childbirth; one in ten women becomes more depressed within the first six weeks or much later; and a tiny minority become very ill.

There are many possible triggers. Labour is stressful, and premature labour especially so. Hormone levels are changing rapidly. And becoming the mother of a new baby causes an emotional upheaval and enormous changes in your life, especially if he needs special care and your life revolves around hospital.

You gain a lot and lose a lot, particularly if you've given up work. And it can take time to start reaping the rewards of motherhood.

It's normal to have mixed feelings but tough if the difficult ones outweigh the positives – as they may, particularly while you're tired and trying to cope with new experiences. However, difficult feelings are better recognised than pushed inside to niggle away and make you depressed.

one in ten women becomes more depressed within the first six weeks

Depression can interfere with sleep, eating, relationships and self-esteem, and trigger panic attacks and obsessional behaviour. Hopefully, this list of tips may help:

- Don't suffer in silence but tell someone how you're feeling. A wise and patient person will listen sensitively and reassure you that although you're feeling horrible, things will improve. They may also steer you towards counselling or drug therapy
- Be kind to yourself by having plenty of rest, frequent meals of good food, daily exercise and half an hour outside each day to get daylight on your skin – in winter preferably at midday
- Ask for all the help you need. Be precise, and give others the jobs you least want. If you need a baby-free break at home, arrange reliable child-care
- Don't even *try* to be a perfect mother. No mother is perfect;

your baby needs only a good enough mother; and you're the tops
- Arrange company if necessary
- Meet other mothers, for example in a parent-and-baby group or – even better – a pre-term parents' group
- Ask about hospital or community groups for women with postnatal depression.

POST-TRAUMATIC STRESS DISORDER

Some women feel stressed and unwell for some time after a premature or difficult birth, or after coping with a very small or ill baby for weeks or months. Besides being anxious and, perhaps, prone to depression or panic attacks, they may have flashbacks, or go off sex because they fear another pregnancy. All this is more likely in women who felt badly informed, ignored or powerless, or who had a lot of pain.

BEREAVEMENT

It's a harsh fact that some babies die. If this happens, the staff will do their utmost to help you and your partner cope with the tragedy and guide the beginning of your journey through your grief.

Your other children will need plenty of help. And your loss will send ripples of sadness among family, friends and neighbours.

Grieving is painful but healing

Take all the time you need with your baby, looking at him, holding him and giving him a name. You might like your baby's photo, cot card, wristband, footprint or lock of hair.

Try not to distance yourself from your feelings unless this is a natural reaction or the only way you can cope at first. Grieving is painful but healing, and helps prevent buried emotions leading later to depression, illness and other signs of post-traumatic stress disorder.

Relationship and sexual difficulties are more likely after a loss, often because the couple can't understand or tolerate each other's reactions. Sensitive listening and an acceptance that each has an individual way of reacting can help.

It's worth seeking all the support you need. The hospital chaplain will offer spiritual support and discuss funeral arrangements. Help is also available from the Stillbirth and Neonatal Death Association. Blisslink/Nippers has a 'Special Memories' group with a newsletter, befrienders' register and support groups. And the Child Bereavement Trust has videos, books and tapes for adults and children (see pp. 176–178 for all).

Many experts recommend avoiding pregnancy for a year or so after losing a baby. This gives a woman and her partner time to come to terms with what's happened and to restore their physical and emotional vitality.

CHAPTER 13

At Home with Your Baby

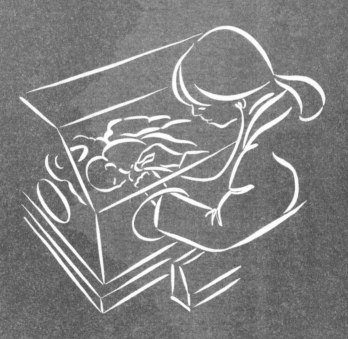

Your baby can come home when she's feeding well, gaining weight steadily and has proved to the SCBU staff that she'll be able to manage. This may be when she's around 36 weeks post-conception age or weighs 1750g (3lb 14oz).

But if she was born before 30 weeks, she may not come home until she's 40 weeks post-conception age or possibly later still.

a baby just out of the SCBU can seem very small and fragile

Most parents, like you, are thrilled to bring their baby home. But a baby just out of the SCBU can seem very small and fragile, and you may feel nervous and have some special concerns. It's perfectly all right to ring the staff at the SCBU if you need information or reassurance.

BREASTFEEDING

Breastfeeding continues to be the best way of nourishing your baby.

Let her feed as often as she wants, but until she's older wake her for a feed if she goes more than four or five hours at night. She'll need night feeds longer than you expect as she has a lot of catching up to do.

She'll spend some time at the breast not actually feeding but just gazing at you and occasionally doing practice-sucking (see p. 57). This boosts your milk supply and can give you some welcome periods of peace and relaxation after your busy, noisy time in hospital.

In the UK a *minimum* of four to six months breastfeeding is officially recommended for all babies. But most babies benefit from much longer. Indeed, the American Academy of Pediatrics recently recommended a minimum of one year of breastfeeding.

However, a premature baby needs to catch up, so should ideally be breastfed for longer than a full-term baby would be. And, of course, you can carry on as long as you and your baby wish.

> *a minimum of four to six months breastfeeding is officially recommended for all babies.*

Help is available from your midwife, health visitor and doctor, and from La Leche League leaders and National Childbirth Trust counsellors (see pp. 177,178).

HOME OXYGEN THERAPY

A few babies need extra oxygen for some time at home (see p. 33). If yours does, the paediatrician will see you regularly and a specially trained nurse may visit. You can get more information from the Blisslink/Nippers leaflet, *Home on Oxygen* (see p. 176).

APNOEA ('STOP-BREATHING') ALARM

Before you leave the SCBU, ask if it would be wise to use an apnoea alarm – a special mattress linked to a monitor – at home.

REDUCING THE RISK OF COT DEATH

There are several easy ways of reducing your baby's risk of cot death:

- For the first few months let her sleep in the same room as you
- Make sure she's warm when she sleeps, but take great care that she doesn't get too hot. You may like to buy a room thermometer and keep the temperature at about 18°C (65°F)
- Tuck the blankets firmly in around her so she's unlikely to wriggle down under them
- Don't use a duvet over or a fleece under your baby for the first year
- Lay her to sleep on her back unless the paediatrician says otherwise
- If she's unwell, contact your doctor without delay
- Don't let her go too long without a breastfeed at night (see above)
- Remember that cigarette smoke is one of the biggest dangers.

SMOKING

Cigarette smoke in the home – from you, your partner or anyone else – makes the sudden infant death syndrome – cot death – more likely. And cot death is more likely anyway in low-birthweight babies, especially very-low-birthweight ones, so it's sensible to be extra careful. Smoking also makes your baby more likely to suffer from asthma and ear and chest infections.

Research shows that lone mothers and mothers whose partner has a semi-skilled or unskilled job, or has no job, are least likely to stop smoking. But if you come into this category, you don't have to become a statistic! Stop-smoking help is available from Quitline (see p. 178).

However, if you can't or don't want to stop:

- Smoke only in another room – and don't take your baby there until you've blown some fresh air through
- Cut down your smoking
- Eat a healthy diet, especially if you're breastfeeding, as having enough nutrients may protect you and your breast-fed baby a little
- Take a multivitamin and mineral supplement especially formulated for nursing mothers if you are breastfeeding.

MASSAGE

Your baby will almost certainly love being massaged. Do it in a warm room, sitting on the floor either with her on a towel on your lap, or with her on a towel on the floor by your side. Use a few drops of baby oil if you like, and stroke her gently and slowly all over.

VISITORS

Don't expose your baby to infections if you can help it. Warn visitors either not to come at all if they have a cold, cough or other infection, or not to go too near or touch her until they're better. This is especially important if you're bottle-feeding. If you're breastfeeding, you needn't be so concerned because your milk helps protect your baby.

LOOKING AFTER YOURSELF

Mothering is rather like being a good manager. And as every manager knows, it's vital to look after yourself so you can enjoy your job and do it well.

So as you settle into being a mother bringing up a premature baby, consider some of the things that might help. Time-management and support are two important issues.

TIME-MANAGEMENT

Premature babies take longer than others to learn the difference between night and day, especially if they've been in an SCBU, and they need frequent feeds for a long time. This means you'll need to juggle frequent feeds and unpredictable sleep and play times, with everything else you do. So you'll have little time to look after yourself unless you work out your priorities and get help with other things.

> *Premature babies take longer than others to learn the difference between night and day*

HELP AND SUPPORT

You may be delighted to accept all the help you can get, or prefer to go it alone, but whatever you do, don't be too proud or shy to ask.

Parents today often don't have the support that past generations did from their extended family living close by. However, support is often available in the community if you need it:

- A great many mothers – and some fathers – enjoy meeting others, swapping experiences, sharing information and, perhaps, campaigning for or even organising improvements in local community facilities. You can do this at a local drop-in club, postnatal group, parent-and-child group, or other women's or parents' groups. Your health visitor or a social worker can tell you about local groups. Blisslink/Nippers (see p. 176) may know of a local one for parents of pre-term babies, but if there isn't one, you might at some stage think of starting one yourself, with their help
- If you'd like to learn more about parenting or would like some support as a parent, contact The Parent Network (see p. 178)
- To discuss a problem with a volunteer, ring Parentline (see p. 178)

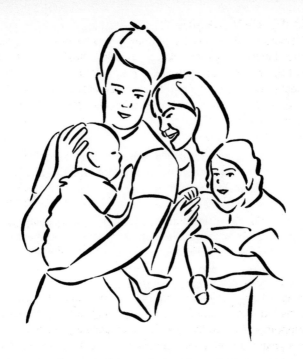

- For a visit from a volunteer 'befriender', contact Homestart (see p. 177)
- Help with health problems is available from your family doctor and health visitor
- Information about rights, benefits and special grants or loans is available from a benefits agency or social worker
- General advice is available from your nearest Citizens' Advice Bureau (address and number in the telephone directory or at the library).

Babysitters. If you go out without your baby, you must leave her with someone you believe to be 100 per cent reliable. A young teenager, however trustworthy and well-meaning, isn't a suitable babysitter for a young baby, especially one who was premature. Give your sitter contact numbers for you, for a neighbour and for the doctor. And if you're breastfeeding, remember you'll need to express milk after and between feeds for several days to leave enough for your sitter to cup-feed your baby while you're out.

WORK

Many people, myself included, believe the most important job the mother of a young child can do is look after that child. And a premature baby needs even more care as she catches up or if she has special needs.

However, increasing numbers of women opt at some stage for the stimulus, financial reward or career-enhancement of a job. They then need the best possible substitute care for their child. Most choose a close family member, while others employ a minder or nanny, or use a nursery.

Each woman has to think through the pros and cons of working in her own personal situation. If you're contemplating going back to work, it may help to write these down and talk them through with your partner or a close friend.

Next we'll look at the likely progress of a low-birthweight baby, as well as the long-term outlook.

CHAPTER 14

Your Baby's Future

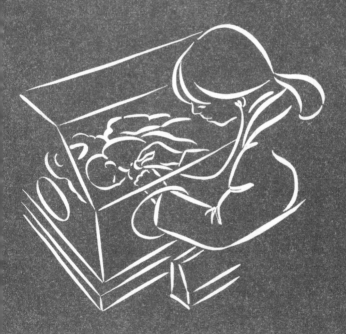

T he vast majority of low-birthweight babies grow healthily and normally.

This chapter gives some broad guidelines on growth and development. It also outlines some possible problems.

Overall, these are very unlikely. So please don't think they happen to every small baby, because they most certainly do not. Also, remember that while every parent wants the best for their child, there's no point comparing your child with any other, because even if they had a similar start, each is an individual and will do things in his own time, at his own rate.

GROWTH

Most low-birthweight babies catch up with their peers in time.

However, very-low-birthweight babies are particularly likely to be smaller than their peers of the same post-conception age for some years. And while most small-for-dates babies do catch up – two out of three in the first six months – some remain small throughout life.

According to a study reported in 1996 of 249 children who were eight years old but with a very low birthweight:

- Eleven out of 12 had caught up size-wise
- Most catching-up was done in the first two years
- Those whose birthweight was appropriate for gestational age were more likely to have caught up than those who were small-for-dates
- The 24 with a serious health or development problem were least likely to have caught up.

Children who had chronic lung disease (broncho-pulmonary dysplasia) as babies are relatively slow to gain weight. Most catch up with their peers in time, but those who were very small at birth or had particularly serious lung problems tend to remain slightly shorter and lighter.

DEVELOPMENT

It helps to count a baby's age from his expected, full-term birthdate, because his developmental skills, such as smiling, sitting, walking and talking, are likely to be delayed by the number of weeks he was premature – and perhaps, if he had a tough time, even longer.

A recent study of children born before 32 weeks and now eight years old found that:

- In those who were small-for-dates, their degree of growth-retardation was related to their intelligence and movement and co-ordination skills
- In those whose birthweight was appropriate for gestational age, their degree of prematurity was related to their movement and co-ordination skills.

ONGOING CONCERNS

The overwhelming majority – nine out of ten premature babies – grow up with no ongoing health or developmental disability. While one in ten does have a persistent problem, this is an *overall* figure

> *nine out of ten premature babies grow up with no ongoing health or developmental disability*

for all premature babies, and the more mature your baby is when he's born, the lower his risk.

For example:

- If born at 32 weeks, his risk of a persistent problem is only one in 50

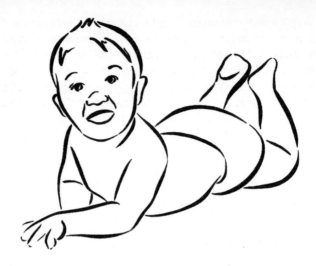

- If born at 28 weeks, his risk of a persistent problem is one in ten
- If born before 26 weeks, surveys put his risk of a persistent significant problem (a severe eyesight or hearing problem, severe learning disability or cerebral palsy) at between one in four and one in ten, though he also has a substantial chance of one or more minor problems. These figures are good news in a way, as they show that 75–90 per cent of surviving babies of this prematurity do *not* have a major ongoing disability. This is much better than a few years ago, when only 60 per cent grew up healthy.

DEVELOPMENTAL PROBLEMS

Regular assessments mean that if your baby is unlucky enough to develop an ongoing problem, he can have help or treatment sooner rather than later.

Differences in intelligence (measured as the IQ) in children who had a low birthweight compared with those whose birthweight was normal are likely to be only small. Studies suggest that those who had a very low birthweight have an average IQ approximately seven points lower than children whose birthweight was normal. One study found that the risk of serious learning difficulty in children who had a very low birthweight was 7–11 times higher than for those of normal weight. And attention deficit disorder (with or without hyperactivity), tics, clumsiness (dyspraxia) and speech difficulty are more common in children who had a low birthweight.

As for cerebral palsy:

- One in two children who develop this condition had a very low birthweight (less than 1500g – 2lb 15oz)
- At least one in 20 very-low-birthweight babies develops cerebral palsy
- The rate of cerebral palsy is perhaps 60–75 times higher in very-low-birthweight babies than in those of normal weight
- Being less than 1000g (1lb 15oz) carries a particularly high risk.

The lower the birthweight, the more likely is an eyesight problem such as short sight, long sight, astigmatism, squint and poor 3-D vision, whether or not a baby develops other visual impairment from retinopathy of prematurity (see p. 98). This makes regular eye checks especially worthwhile.

Hearing problems are also more likely in low-birthweight babies, especially very-low-birthweight ones, and regular hearing tests – starting soon after birth – are an excellent idea.

A young child who was very premature may have mottled or yellowish teeth.

HEALTH PROBLEMS

IN CHILDHOOD

One large study of low-birthweight babies found that by the age of two, those whose birthweight was appropriate for gestational age had a higher risk of asthma, wheezing and higher blood pressure than those who'd been small-for-dates. So prematurity seemed a bigger risk than growth-retardation.

The lungs of babies with chronic lung disease continue to heal, though in the early months these babies may be more 'chesty' or wheezy with each cough or cold.

IN ADULT LIFE

Being born short, thin and small-for-dates makes non-insulin-dependent (type 2) diabetes and cardiovascular disease (high blood pressure, coronary heart disease and strokes) more likely – but seemingly only in those adults who become overweight. Adults born prematurely *and* small-for-dates have a particularly high risk. And a low birthweight appears to double the risk of coronary heart disease.

Some researchers have suggested that the link could be certain types of undernourishment of a pregnant woman – and hence, undernourishment of her baby – at certain crucial times of pregnancy. However, other experts hotly dispute this and point out that the evidence is based on retrospective epidemiological studies – population studies which look backward and 'prove' very little.

No one yet knows how undernourishment in pregnancy might affect the cardiovascular system of the unborn baby, but some experts suggest it could:

• Prevent elastin deposition in the baby's artery walls, making them less elastic and so encouraging cardiovascular disease in adult life, especially if overweight. (If this does indeed happen, I wonder whether the reason why a woman born with a low birthweight is more likely to give birth prematurely herself – see p. 134 – is because she has inelastic womb arteries.) Elastin is made of extremely long-lived molecules – it's 'half-life' (the time it takes for 50 per cent to be destroyed) is 40 years! And virtually none of an adult's elastin is replaced. So the elastin a baby lays down could be most important for future health

- Weaken the heart's left ventricle (lower left chamber) by back pressure as blood is diverted from the aorta (the big artery from the heart) to the brain to try to prevent a shortage of blood – and essential nutrients – to this vital organ
- Programme a baby's metabolism to deal differently with insulin and glucose, raising the risk of diabetes, heart disease and strokes.

Other research is investigating whether small-for-dates babies either have abnormally low levels of insulin (and, as a result, low levels of growth hormone and insulin-like growth factor) or abnormally high levels of insulin (and growth hormone). If so, this could either mean that undernourishment in the womb affected the baby's pancreas, or that it was already defective.

If you have a small-for-dates baby, it makes sense to encourage lifestyle habits in your family which may minimise his risk of being unhealthily overweight in years to come.

If you have a small-for-dates baby, it makes sense to encourage lifestyle habits in your family which may minimise his risk of being unhealthily overweight in years to come. Such habits include a healthy diet and a daily half-hour's exercise.

There are also associations between low birthweight and, as an adult:

- 'Apple-shaped' obesity – fat stored around the waist – the sort of fatness linked with a higher risk of 'insulin resistance' diabetes (the non-insulin-dependent type) and heart disease. Insulin resistance may develop into diabetes during pregnancy (see p. 167)
- A raised risk of having a stillborn baby or one who dies soon after birth. One study found this risk was doubled if the

woman's birthweight was 1500–2000g (3lb 5oz–4lb 6oz) and trebled if under 1500g
- Chronic bronchitis and emphysema
- A lower bone mineral content and a higher risk of osteoporosis.
- Women who as unborn babies suffered from growth-retardation in the womb are more likely to have pre-eclampsia when they themselves become pregnant.

And in adults who were low-birthweight babies and still small for their age at one year, researchers have found earlier signs of ageing than in their normal birthweight peers, with:
- More likelihood of cataract
- Worse hearing
- Reduced grip strength
- Thinner skin.

One fascinating theory is that undernourishment in the womb prevents the normal amount of certain long-lived molecules being laid down in that unborn baby's body. Such molecules include elastin in artery walls (see above), collagen in the inner ear, collagen and elastin in muscle and crystallins in the lenses of the eyes.

SURVIVAL

Thanks to medical technology the survival of babies born after 25 weeks has improved dramatically over the last two decades. However, life is still extremely risky for 23- or 24-week-old babies, and only a handful of 22-week-olds have ever survived.

Each extra week in the womb makes a big difference – with babies born after 36 weeks being 50 times more likely to live than the very smallest

the survival of babies born after 25 weeks has improved dramatically

prems. At 23 weeks, 16 per cent of babies survive, and at 26 weeks, 57 per cent. At 28 weeks, the brain and other organs are sufficiently well developed for there to be a good chance of survival. And over 30 weeks, getting on for 100 per cent survive.

The length of pregnancy isn't such a reliable indicator for a small-for-dates baby's chance of survival, because he's had to cope with undernourishment in the womb. However, in developed countries such as the UK, prematurity is a bigger problem in terms of survival than is being small-for-dates.

- Overall, one in ten babies born before 37 weeks dies, with the youngest, lightest, shortest and thinnest the least likely to survive.
- Over nine out of ten babies born at 28 weeks can now survive. And while a few years ago only a small percentage of those babies born at 27 weeks pulled through, seven out of ten now live.
- More than one in three (35 per cent) babies born at 25 weeks survives overall, and over half those reaching a neonatal intensive care unit (NICU) survive.
- Up to 42 in 100 babies born at 24 weeks and reaching a NICU survive. A short time ago, baby Jordan Smith was born in Florida at just over 24 weeks. She weighed in at only 700g (1lb 6oz), her foot was just over one and a half times the length of an old 50 pence piece, and her hand was little larger than her father's thumbnail.
- Although overall only five in every 100 babies born at 23 weeks survive, over 27 in 100 reaching a NICU do so; the lucky survivors have a chance of surviving normal, bright and unscathed.

The question that springs to mind now is what causes prematurity and growth retardation in the first place?

CHAPTER 15

Why Are Some Babies Born So Early and So Small?

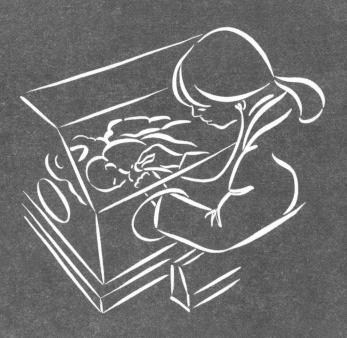

Docters arrange one in three premature births. The rest are spontaneous and half the time there's no obvious trigger.

As with growth-retardation, only sometimes is the reason for premature birth completely clear.

WHAT'S NEEDED FOR LABOUR TO START?

Researchers are still working out what combination of factors makes the womb expel a baby – or a baby bid farewell to the womb.

Several mechanisms which help prime the womb for labour are becoming clearer, including:

CERVIX RIPENING

The coil of strong, inelastic collagen fibres in the cervix is normally stuck together by glycoprotein 'glue', but early in labour this glue becomes less sticky. The cervix becomes waterlogged. It also becomes shorter and adopts a funnel shape. Early softening, shortening and 'ripening' lead to premature labour; the triggers may include the balance of hormones, the presence of fetal fibronectin (see p. 173), and the levels of nitric oxide and inflammatory chemicals called cytokines.

ENHANCED WOMB CONTRACTILITY

Several things make contractions more likely, including:
• Changing hormone levels (oestrogen, oestrogen–proges-terone ratio, corticotrophin-releasing hormone, oxytocin,

relaxin and adrenaline)

- Levels of certain prostaglandins – hormone-like substances which can make the womb muscles more likely to tighten up.
- Neurotransmitter levels (serotonin and acetylcholine)
- Levels of other substances (including endorphins, nitric oxide and platelet-activating factor).

These factors act either by altering the calcium ion concentration in womb muscle cells or the sensitivity of these cells to calcium. The acidity (pH) of the cells is probably important only in prolonged labour, when the muscle becomes more acid and contracts less easily.

ACTIVATION OF FREQUENT, CO-ORDINATED CONTRACTIONS

The heavily pregnant womb often has 'practice' (Braxton Hicks) contractions, but to begin the frequent, highly co-ordinated contractions of labour it must first be 'activated'. Part of this activation is a rise in the number of womb receptors for certain contraction-encouraging substances. This rise is probably controlled by oestrogen, progesterone and the degree of stretch in the womb.

PLACENTAL CLOCK

The 'clock' which determines when labour begins may be an interaction between oxytocin and the corticotrophin-releasing hormone.

WHAT ENCOURAGES PREMATURE LABOUR AND GROWTH-RETARDATION?

Many lifestyle factors and health problems contribute to a baby's risk of being premature or small-for-dates. Let's take them in turn.

AN UNHEALTHY PLACENTA

If the placenta doesn't perform properly, a baby doesn't get enough nourishment and won't grow well. She may also have insufficient oxygen and become distressed, making an early birth essential. This 'placental insufficiency' can develop if the mother smokes, eats poorly, drinks a lot of alcohol, or has an infection, high blood pressure, or Hughes' syndrome. It may also be more likely if she herself was a growth-retarded baby. And sometimes there's no obvious reason.

Researchers are investigating several possible problems underlying an unhealthy placenta:

- A lack of growth factors – or their receptors – in the placenta
- A high rate of cell death ('programmed' cell death or apoptosis) in the placenta or membranes
- A poor blood flow to the placenta because of failure of the artery supplying the womb to widen when necessary in response to natural substances such as nitric oxide
- A poor blood flow to the placenta due to its blood vessels not linking properly with those in the wall of the womb.

HIGH BLOOD PRESSURE

High blood pressure in the mother can make the placenta unhealthy and may result from:

- Simple pregnancy-induced high blood pressure
- Pre-existing high blood pressure, for example from previous kidney disease
- Pre-eclampsia – see below.

PRE-ECLAMPSIA

Researchers believe that pre-eclampsia – high blood pressure plus leaking of protein from the kidneys into the urine, heralding the possibility of fits (eclampsia) – may result partly from minute bits of placenta entering the mother's bloodstream and preventing her arteries from widening when necessary.

Pre-eclampsia is more likely in women with:
- A raised risk of high blood pressure unrelated to pregnancy
- A raised risk of insulin resistance (high levels of insulin after eating certain carbohydrates, refined ones in particular) and diabetes
- A history of being a growth-retarded baby (see p. 27)
- A mother or sister who had pre-eclampsia
- A short relationship with the baby's father before conception. The shorter this is, the higher the risk of pre-eclampsia. But a long relationship is protective only if neither condoms nor a diaphragm are used. A woman who hasn't cohabited throughout a long relationship loses some of its protection, so perhaps the more her cervix is exposed to her partner's semen, the

> *Pre-eclampsia is usually most severe in a first pregnancy*

greater her chance of becoming immune to his genes or whatever else in semen may decrease her risk of pre-eclampsia. For it's possible, though unproven, that a woman's immune system reacts as if her baby were 'foreign' – which, of course, she partly is. Pre-eclampsia is usually most severe in a first pregnancy. However, if a woman then has a baby by another man – meaning her immune system has to deal with another man's genes – her pre-eclampsia may not be less this time, or may develop for the first time.

Treatment is with rest and early delivery if necessary to protect mother or baby. Daily low-dose aspirin benefits only a few women with symptoms before 32 weeks.

Researchers are investigating whether taking vitamins C and E each day could minimise or prevent pre-eclampsia in high-risk women. They think that free radicals produced in an unhealthy placenta can damage blood vessels throughout the body and cause high blood pressure. The anti-oxidant action of these vitamins might mop up these free radicals and prevent damage.

POOR DIET

This is one of the easiest factors to remedy.

You have a greater chance of having a premature or growth-retarded baby if you are:

- Underweight before you conceive
- Poorly nourished before you conceive
- Poorly nourished in pregnancy – deficiencies of calcium, iron, magnesium, zinc, flavonoids (plant pigments in vegetables and fruits), vitamin B and essential fatty acids (certain polyunsaturated fatty acids) are linked with low birthweight
- Eat too much (more than 340 grams) carbohydrate each day
- Put on too little weight when pregnant.

Most pregnant women know what they need, though some don't eat properly and a few don't eat enough good food in a misguided attempt to avoid putting on too much weight. But a major reason for eating badly in pregnancy is poverty.

A Maternity Alliance survey (1995) showed that some pregnant women in the UK on state benefits didn't have enough money to eat a nutritionally adequate diet which was culturally acceptable and attractive enough for them to want. The researchers were especially concerned about pregnant 16- and 17-year-olds; they need a particularly nutritious diet because they are themselves growing.

This is a terrible situation and we should be ashamed of ourselves as a nation for allowing it to continue. The Maternity Alliance (see p. 177) has made recommendations to the government in *Poor Expectations: Poverty and Undernourishment in Pregnancy*.

A good diet for men and women supplies anti-mutagenic nutrients which help protect sperms, eggs and embryo from genetic damage (see below). These include beta-carotene (a vitamin A-like substance in fruits and vegetables), vitamins B,

C and E, selenium, zinc, polyunsaturated fatty acids (needed to make DHA, below), mono-unsaturated fatty acids and chlorophyll (a pigment in green leafy vegetables).

However, the Maternity Alliance survey found one in five women on benefits had a serious deficiency of one or more of the following – vitamins A, B and C, calcium, iron, magnesium and potassium.

And if money is tight, then rather than give their men insufficient food many women go short themselves. So having too little good food is most likely to be a woman's problem.

Other research reveals that one in ten unborn babies risks growth-retardation from too little DHA (the fatty acid docosahexaenoic acid). This may result from the mother being unable to make enough in her body because her diet lacks enough of the omega 3 polyunsaturated fatty acids that are the building blocks for DHA.

HAVING BABIES CLOSE TOGETHER

This can reduce a baby's birthweight if a woman has not had enough time – or a good enough diet – to replenish her body's nutrient stores between pregnancies. The optimal spacing is considered to be over two to four years.

optimal spacing is considered to be over two to four years

TOO MUCH ALCOHOL

Too much alcohol in pregnancy (the regular consumption of at least two units a day) can lead to the fetal alcohol syndrome, with low birthweight, a particular appearance (small head, short nose and thin lips), defects such as a hole in the heart or spinal abnormality, and severe learning difficulties.

AN UNDERACTIVE THYROID GLAND

Untreated, this makes pre-term birth more likely.

PLANNED OR EMERGENCY PREMATURE DELIVERY

Doctors arrange one in three premature births for the safety of mother or baby.

Examples of situations sometimes or always needing elective (planned) or emergency delivery include:

- A shortage of oxygen
- Poor or no growth
- Rhesus disease
- High blood pressure in the mother
- Diabetes in the mother
- Prematurely ruptured membranes with evidence of infection
- Placenta praevia – a placenta attached too low in the womb, against the cervix – as this can lead to bleeding
- Bleeding from the placenta as it separates prematurely from the wall of the womb (placental 'abruption').

PREMATURE RUPTURE OF THE MEMBRANES

Up to one in two premature births begins with spontaneous rupture of the amniotic membranes, though this is rare before 26 weeks.

During pregnancy the maternal and fetal membranes are glued together with a protein called **fibronectin**. They start breaking down some weeks before labour, thereby freeing fibronectin.

Finding fibronectin in the vagina after 20 weeks suggests that the membranes are already breaking down and may rupture early. A positive fibronectin test (currently under evaluation in the UK, see p. 173) is currently the most powerful predictor of spontaneous premature labour.

Premature rupture may result from:

- An infection in the vagina (see below) reaching the womb and weakening the membranes
- Other problems making the membranes weak
- The cervix dilating too soon

- Twins or more
- Medical procedures such as amniocentesis
- No obvious cause.

INFECTION
Several infections in the mother may encourage premature labour or growth-retardation, or both:

- **Bacteria from the vagina**. Bacteria can travel to the womb from a vaginal infection (such as gonorrhoea, or chlamydia infection), or from a vaginal overgrowth of bacteria which are normally present but usually harmless (bacterial vaginosis, see above and p.137 and p. 151). These organisms may then inflame the womb's membranes (chorioamnionitis). Researchers believe this not only makes premature rupture of the membranes more likely (see above), but can also trigger premature labour by increasing the concentration of certain prostaglandins (hormone-like substances that encourage womb contractions). Some reports suggest that a vaginal infection or overgrowth in early pregnancy doubles the risk of late miscarriage or premature birth; others that it multiplies the risk sixfold. It's wise to treat vaginal infection in pregnancy. The small amount of research to date from the US suggests it may be wise to treat bacterial overgrowth as well – but only in women who have a high risk of having a premature baby, such as those who have given birth prematurely before. Unfortunately, one in two affected women doesn't know she has a potential problem, or thinks her vaginal discharge is thrush and uses the wrong treatment
- **Flu, rubella** (see p. 151) **and certain other viral infections**
- **Urine infection** can cause a high fever and trigger premature labour
- **Toxoplasmosis** (see p. 152)
- **Listeriosis** (see p. 152) can lead to miscarriage, stillbirth or premature labour
- **Gum disease** (see p. 151). It's suggested that gum disease

accounts for more than one in six premature births (which makes it more risky than smoking or alcohol!) and that severe gum disease raises the risk of prematurity 7.5 times. Researchers postulate that bacteria or their toxins from diseased gums travel in the blood to the womb, where they damage the placenta. These bacteria or toxins also stimulate a woman's body to make inflammatory chemicals which can trigger

> *gum disease accounts for more than one in six premature births*

labour. If further studies prove this is so, I expect the problem may be worse if a dentist or dental hygienist disturbs sore gums. After all, even eating an apple or brushing the teeth can release bacteria from diseased gums into the bloodstream.

SMOKING

Smoking – especially in the second half of pregnancy – increases the risk of a difficult birth, makes the placenta unhealthy and raises a baby's risk of being growth-retarded and premature. The average reduction in birthweight is 200g (8oz) – which is a lot, particularly if other problems reduce the birthweight, too.

Smoking probably lowers a baby's future intelligence and raises her risk of infections, cot death and perhaps leukaemia. *And the lower a baby's birthweight, the higher her risk of serious ill health and permanent disability in childhood and adult life.*

Passive smoking is a problem, too. In 1997 US researchers reported that passive smoking made non-smoking women over 30 more likely to have premature and low-birthweight babies.

Smoking can make the placenta separate from the womb (placental abruption) and lead to premature labour. And it raises a woman's blood cadmium level. This heavy metal then lowers her level of zinc – a metal which is an essential nutrient for normal fetal growth.

ANTIPHOSPHOLIPID SYNDROME (see also p. 174)
Some women have antiphospholipid antibodies which cause small blood clots in the placenta. This encourages miscarriage, pre-eclampsia, growth-retardation and premature birth. And it's more common in women with kidney disease due to lupus (systemic lupus erythematosus), an auto-immune disorder .

MULTIPLES
Twins, triplets or more increase the chance of delivering early, because multiple babies stretch the womb and make the membranes more likely to rupture early. Quads are generally born at around 31 weeks, triplets at 33, and twins later. The average birthweight of a triplet is 1800g (3lb 15oz), and a twin 2500g (5lb 8oz).

Fertility treatment makes multiple conception more likely. The last decade and a half in the UK has witnessed a big increase in assisted conception and fertility drug treatment, and a corresponding increase in multiple births – especially triplets or more. At least one in ten very-low-birthweight babies is conceived after fertility treatment.

LOW FERTILITY
Not only does fertility treatment make multiple birth and low birthweight more likely, but also women who report difficulty in conceiving but don't have fertility treatment are more likely to have a low-birthweight baby.

PREVIOUS PREMATURE OR
LOW-BIRTHWEIGHT BABY
Most women who've had a premature or other low-birth-

weight baby for no obvious reason have a full-term one next time. However, your risk of another premature baby is five times that of a woman who hasn't had one, giving you a one in six chance. And if you've had two previous low-birthweight, premature babies, your risk of another rises to one in three.

PREVIOUS ABORTION
Two or more abortions make subsequent births more likely to be premature.

AN UNUSUALLY SHAPED WOMB
This sometimes expels a fetus before 37 weeks.

FIBROIDS
It's possible, though unusual, for a uterine fibroid to retard a baby's growth. A fibroid can also make the placenta separate from the womb (placental abruption) and bleed, leading to premature labour or an emergency Caesarean.

TOO MUCH OR TOO LITTLE AMNIOTIC FLUID
Either of these may result in premature labour. Maternal diabetes, multiple babies or an abnormality in the baby sometimes causes too much fluid. An abnormal placenta, pre-eclampsia or a kidney problem in the baby sometimes causes too little.

RHESUS DISEASE (see pp. 45 and 174)

One recent study found that working long hours when pregnant reduces a baby's growth by an average of 80g (under 3oz). Work involving lifting, prolonged standing and climbing did not affect fetal growth. However, the babies of women who combined long working hours with physically demanding work were up to 350g (10oz) lighter than expected. Other studies have found that either heavy work or standing a lot can increase the risk of having a low-birthweight baby. One large study found that working more than 40 hours a week in a mentally demanding profession increased the risk of having a premature baby by 70%! And feeling powerless at work is another big risk factor.

STRESS

A severe shock raises the risk of having a miscarriage. And a large US study of 2593 pregnant women found that those who were stressed were more likely to have a pre-term or low-birth-weight baby. They were also more likely to smoke, which added to the problem.

USE OF THE PILL OR COPPER COIL

If a woman uses the Pill or copper coil until just before conception, high levels of copper and low levels of zinc may encourage prematurity.

DRUG USE

Women who use cannabis regularly seem more likely to have a low-birthweight baby. If a woman regularly takes cannabis and alcohol (see p. 160), her baby may also have a higher chance of the fetal alcohol syndrome. Cocaine is thought to make prematurity more likely. And amphetamines raise the risk of a baby being pre-term and/or growth-retarded.

LEAD EXPOSURE

Lead exposure can reduce a woman's zinc level and lead to her baby having a low birthweight. This may happen from:
- Careless stripping of lead-containing paint (see p. 154)
- Using lead-containing Indian cosmetics
- Prolonged exposure to traffic fumes
- Consuming lead-polluted food or water.

CADMIUM EXPOSURE

Cadmium exposure has been linked to low birthweight.
    This may happen from:
- Smoking
- Using cadmium-containing art pigments (certain reds and yellows)
- Exposure to certain pesticides
- Consuming certain refined cereals, tinned food and water.

GIRL BABY

Girls have a higher risk of a low birthweight than boys, though low-birthweight girls are more likely to survive. The average full-term boy weighs 140g (5oz) more than the average full-term girl.

BIRTH ORDER

The average second full-term baby is 100g (4oz) heavier than the average first full-term one. So a firstborn has a slightly higher chance of a low birthweight.

ABNORMALITY

A genetic or other abnormality makes a low birthweight more likely.
    Factors encouraging an abnormality include exposure of sperm or egg before pregnancy, or exposure of a very newly conceived embryo to:
- X-rays
- Pesticides
- Burning plastics
- Vapour from solvents (such as perchloroethylene, used by dry-cleaners), glues etc.
- Chemicals at work.

BEING UNDER 16

Very young mothers are less likely to carry their babies to term. One US survey found that young adolescents were 75 per cent

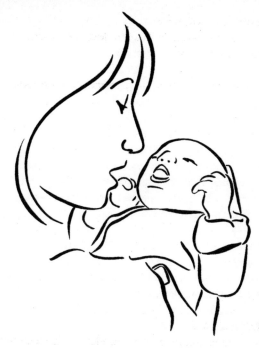

more likely to have a pre-term labour. The risk was highest in those who began having periods less than two years before their pregnancy.

POVERTY

The majority of low-birthweight babies in western countries are born to low-income women. In the UK one in three is born into a family living in poverty (a household receiving means-tested state benefits, or with an income of less than half the national average). There's recently been a big increase in the number of children living in poverty in the UK and each day another 600 babies join the very poor.

These alarming statistics result from financially disadvan-taged women being:

- More likely to have a baby when under 16
- More likely to smoke or live with a smoker
- More likely to have a tiring job involving hard physical labour and to be on their feet a lot
- More likely to be unwell and, perhaps, to have infections
- Less likely to have a nutritious diet (see above).

DOMESTIC VIOLENCE

Between 2 per cent and 20 per cent of women seen in antenatal clinics have experienced severe physical, emotional or sexual violence. And physical violence – especially if directed at a woman's abdomen – makes miscarriage, prematurity and low birthweight more likely.

FOOD ALLERGY AND INTOLERANCE?

I've looked unsuccessfully for published research demonstrating any link, or lack of it, between food allergy and prematurity or growth-retardation. However, I found one study which reported that women with coeliac disease (intolerance to the cereal protein gluten in wheat, barley, rye and oats) were more prone to miscarriage. This might be an area worth researching further.

Some things which make babies premature or small-for-dates are clearly the responsibility of a civilised society. But the next chapter looks at what you yourself can do before you get pregnant again to lower your risk of having another low-birthweight baby.

CHAPTER 16

Thinking About Having Another Baby?

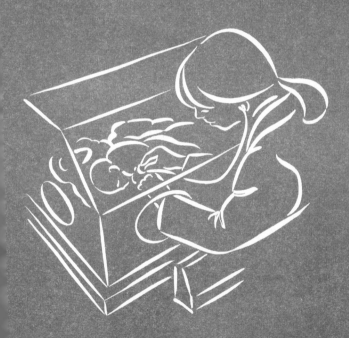

A pre-conception health and fitness programme makes sperm and eggs more likely to be healthy. It also encourages a healthy, full-term pregnancy. And the best time to start is before you stop using contraception.

There's certainly no guarantee that doing this will prevent you having another low-birthweight baby, but it just might. And anyway, it won't do you or your next baby any harm and will probably make you feel better!

EATING WELL

Eating nutrient-packed food helps you maintain a healthy weight, fills your nutrient stores and gets you into the habit of eating well in good time for pregnancy. This is important because a baby's weight is partly programmed very early in pregnancy. One study found that mothers of low-birthweight babies were much more likely than others to have eaten a nutrient-poor diet in pregnancy; their nutrient deficit around conception was especially striking.

So go for:
- Five or more daily helpings of salad, fruit and vegetables. A 'helping' is a small bowlful, or a piece of fruit
- Foods rich in folic acid (green leafy vegetables, citrus fruit, beans, peas, potatoes, oranges, fortified bread and cereal, nuts and Marmite)
- Two helpings a day of meat, fish, eggs, beans or peas
- Nuts, seeds and lentils
- Cold-pressed oils (such as olive and walnut oils, and unre-

fined sunflower oil from health food shops) for salad dressings
- Oily fish (such as sardines, pilchards, herrings, kippers, salmon, etc.) three times a week
- Four daily portions of bread, pasta, rice, potatoes or cereals. Choose some wholegrain foods (wholemeal bread, wholegrain breakfast cereals and brown rice) rather than only foods made from refined grains (white bread, rice and pasta, many breakfast cereals, and cakes, biscuits and pastry made with white flour)
- Not too many foods containing added sugar
- Not too much animal and other largely saturated fat (butter, margarine and other hard cooking and spreading fats, cakes, biscuits, pastry, fried foods, crisps and many other manufactured snacks, and most types of red meat).

Most people are fairly clear about healthy eating, but if you'd like to know more or discuss ideas, for example, about shopping and cooking on a tight budget, ask your health visitor. She may also know of a cookery club in your area, or a course or centre which provides opportunities to meet others and discuss ideas.

FOLIC ACID SUPPLEMENTS

A daily folic acid supplement is an excellent idea. Ask your doctor for a prescription and begin taking it from a month before you intend starting to try for a baby. Continue for at least the first 12 weeks of pregnancy.
- A woman planning her first baby needs a 400mcg (micrograms) tablet of folic acid each day.
- A woman who has previously miscarried a baby with a neural tube defect (or lost such a baby) needs a ten times higher dose of 4mg (milligrams).

OTHER SUPPLEMENTS

It's especially sensible to take other supplements if you or your partner:
- Eats an unhealthy diet
- Is underweight because of eating too little
- Continues to smoke
- Drinks more than a little
- Has fertility problems.
  Or if you:
- Have had a miscarriage, pre-term baby or stillborn baby before
- Had a baby in the last year
- Have had pre-eclampsia before.

For you: a daily, multivitamin and mineral supplement formulated especially for pre-conception and pregnancy, and a supplement of the fatty acid DHA (docosahexaenoic acid). Your baby's need for DHA is most marked after six months of pregnancy, when the brain is growing very fast. Ask your pharmacist which brands to buy; you needn't take folic acid separately because a pregnancy multivitamin and mineral supplement contains the recommended amount.

For your partner: any multipurpose, multivitamin and mineral supplement.

YOUR WEIGHT

If you're underweight or overweight, try to achieve and maintain a healthy weight as far ahead of starting a baby as possible; if you diet, stop dieting at least three months before you try for a baby.

This takes time and effort but is important because:
- Being underweight before you conceive increases your risk

of having a low-birthweight baby

- Being overweight when pregnant increases your risk of high blood pressure (especially if you were a small-for-dates baby), which increases your baby's risk of growth-retardation
- A good nutrient supply helps prevent your baby being malformed and miscarried, and helps you feel well.

try to achieve and maintain a healthy weight as far ahead of starting a baby as possible

EXERCISE

Almost everyone feels better if they get their body moving and their hearts and lungs working faster for at least half an hour a day. Their weight tends to stabilise at a healthy level. They feel happier and are more likely to keep well. And now's the time to start doing it.

Exercise boosts the circulation and is good news for carrying a baby successfully.

If you yourself were born small-for-dates and are over-weight, regular exercise is particularly important as this will help you shed your excess weight before you get pregnant. And if you're extremely overweight, then whatever your own birthweight, daily exercise will help prevent diabetes developing in pregnancy.

DAYLIGHT

Spend time outside each day to get daylight on your skin. Even in northern latitudes the light you absorb even just through your face will help. Top up your light exposure in the summer and if, in winter, you can spare only a little time, go outside at midday.

Having sufficient light:

- Boosts oestrogen – necessary for a healthy, full-term pregnancy
- Helps relieve stress by preventing winter depression (seasonal affective disorder or SAD).

SMOKING AND PASSIVE SMOKING

If you smoke, it's best to stop or, at the very least, cut right down at least three months before trying for a baby.

Handling and smoking cigarettes and inhaling nicotine may be temporarily relaxing and comforting – and you may think it's 'cool' – but it's detrimental to your unborn baby's growth and health (see p.138 and p. 158).

Tips on stopping are available from Quitline (see p. 178); a special Quitline for pregnant women may at some stage become nationally available. If your partner also smokes, you are most likely to give up if he does too.

If you can't stop or decide not to, at least eat a healthy diet; smokers tend to have less nutritious diets than non-smokers do – another thing that disadvantages their babies.

STRESS

A certain amount of stress is stimulating. Sometimes, though, stress becomes too much to handle. It isn't always possible to reduce the stresses in life, but if you'd like to learn to handle them more effectively, it may pay to read a book on the subject, go on a stress-management course or consult a counsellor. And don't forget to ask for as much backup as you need from friends and family.

Domestic violence is one important cause of stress often ignored by embarrassed, helpless outsiders and kept quiet by victims and perpetrators. If a man physically damages his partner before she gets pregnant, the likelihood is he'll do it again when she's pregnant. And some men are violent for the first time when their partner is pregnant. *For this reason, and because ongoing violence is unacceptable, it's essential to get help now* by confiding in your health visitor, doctor or social worker, or by ringing the Women's Aid National Helpline on 0345 023 468.

RUBELLA IMMUNISATION

Rubella (German measles) in pregnancy can increase the risk of low birthweight, so if you've never been immunised, ask your doctor for a blood test to see if you're immune. If you're not, you can be immunised – but it's crucial not to get pregnant for a month afterwards.

INFECTIONS

Steer clear, if you can, of children and adults who are unwell and either have or are expecting to get flu, chickenpox or other common infections.

GUM DISEASE

Look after your teeth and gums with a healthy diet, daily brushing and flossing, and regular visits to the dentist. A new blood test reveals that as many as 30 per cent of people carry a 'gum disease' gene, making their risk of gum disease up to 18 times higher. If you have gum disease, get it treated now.

VAGINAL INFECTION OR BACTERIAL OVER-GROWTH (see p. 137)

This sometimes leads to womb infection and encourages premature labour, so ask for your doctor's advice if you have a discharge or other vaginal symptoms. Some women regularly douche to 'clean' their vaginas, but this disturbs the normal balance of organisms and is best avoided.

If your partner has a discharge from his penis, or other

symptoms which may suggest non-gonococcal urethritis (inflammation of the urethra – the urine passage), he should see his doctor for treatment; otherwise you could pass bacteria between you each time you have sex.

LISTERIOSIS
Since you could become pregnant any time, take care not to eat:
1 Pâté made from meat, fish or vegetables
2 Blue-veined or mould-ripened cheeses (such as Brie and Camembert). Experts in the US also warn against feta cheese
3 Soft-whip ice cream
4 Unpasteurised milk
5 Pre-cooked poultry
6 Cooked chilled food – unless thoroughly reheated
7 Prepared salads – unless thoroughly washed
8 Underdone meat.

TOXOPLASMOSIS
Getting toxoplasmosis in pregnancy can damage a woman's baby and lead to prematurity.
   So help prevent it by:
1 Wearing rubber gloves when handling soil
2 Washing salads, vegetables and fruit before eating
3 Avoiding raw or undercooked meat
4 Washing your hands after handling raw meat
5 Wearing rubber gloves to empty your cat's litter tray – or getting someone else to do it
6 Disinfecting the litter tray each day with boiling water
7 Avoiding contact with sick cats.

MEDICATION

Avoid any medication unless you have checked with your doctor or pharmacist that it is safe when trying for a baby or in early pregnancy.

ENVIRONMENTAL HAZARDS

X-RAYS

If you need an X-ray, tell the person doing it that you're thinking of getting pregnant – in case you already are! A non-emergency X-ray is best scheduled for the first week of your menstrual cycle and you must be sure to wear extra radiation protection, such as a lead apron.

PESTICIDES

Exposure to biocides – weedkillers (herbicides) and pesticides (insecticides and fungicides) – may endanger eggs and sperm and damage or kill unborn babies. Any poisonous household, garden, pet or agricultural biocide should carry prominent warnings and instructions. Unless you're sure it's safe, don't inhale biocide vapour, and keep the chemical off your skin.

If you live within a quarter of a mile of crops being sprayed, go away for the day unless you know the product is a harmless fertiliser or a biocide not dangerous to humans. Afterwards, avoid walking near newly sprayed fields and inhaling mist hanging over them.

Wash, scrub or peel salads, vegetables and fruit to remove pesticide traces, or eat organic produce. A Soil Association spokesman says: '...it's impossible to protect consumers from organophosphate residues simply by requiring growers to use pesticides more carefully.'

BURNING PLASTICS
Avoid breathing smoke from burning plastics; if these contain PVC (polyvinylchloride), their smoke may contain dangerous PCBs (polychlorinated biphenyls).

VAPOUR FROM SOLVENTS, GLUES, ETC.
Avoid inhaling vapour from solvents, paints, thinners, glues and marking pens.

LEAD (see p. 141)
Try, if you can, to avoid too much exposure to sources of environmental lead. Any stripping of lead paint should be done very carefully by someone else and you should keep well away (see *How to Remove Old Lead Paint* leaflet, p. 179).

CADMIUM (see p. 141)
Avoid overexposure to cadmium.

CHEMICALS AT WORK
If you work with chemicals, check that your employer carries out any necessary safety precautions for women who might be – or already are – pregnant. Some potentially hazardous chemicals are mentioned above; others include mercury, cytotoxic drugs, perchlorethylene, ethylene glycol esters, formaldehyde, glutaraldehyde and anaesthetic gases. The highest risks are in the chemical, plastics, pharmaceutical, rubber and textile industries, as well as in market gardening, dry-cleaning and farming.

WHEN TO COME OFF THE PILL OR HAVE A COIL OUT (see p. 141)

THE PILL
Ideally, stop the Pill at least three months (and some experts recommend up to 12) before you want to conceive. An added

advantage of doing this is that you have a better chance of restoring regular periods before you get pregnant, which will make dating your baby's age easier.

In the meantime use a condom, diaphragm or the sympto-thermal method (perhaps with the help of a saliva microscope or electronic ovulation monitor). Your doctor will give you more information.

THE COIL
Have a copper coil removed six months before you want to get pregnant.

FERTILITY TREATMENT

If you need fertility treatment, the doctors will do their best to ensure you carry no more than one or, at the most, two babies. However, sometimes a newly fertilised egg splits into two, forming twins, and many women have a better chance of successful pregnancy if they start with more than one embryo.

Treatments sometimes associated with more than one fetus include:
- Hormone therapy to stimulate egg release (superovulation)
- IVF-ET (*in vitro* fertilisation plus embryo transfer) – surgical removal of eggs and subsequent fertilisation with the part-ner's sperm in a test tube and transfer of one or more embryos to the woman's cervix or womb
- GIFT (gamete intra-Fallopian transfer) – surgical removal of eggs, which are mixed with the partner's sperm and put into a Fallopian tube
- Donor IVF – mixing donated eggs from another woman with the partner's sperm, then putting them in the infertile woman's womb.

DRUGS

If you're a drug user, look after yourself and your baby by coming off them. Help is available from the National Drugs Helpline on 0800 77 66 00.

Continue your pre-conception health programme until you're pregnant and then on into pregnancy.

CHAPTER 17

Pregnant Again

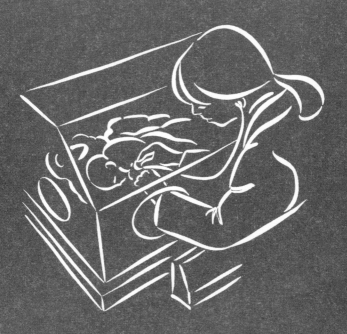

W hen you get pregnant, carry on caring for yourself as described in the last chapter. This 'peri-conceptual care' – care before and after conception – makes you as healthy as possible and protects your baby from the very beginning – before you realise you're pregnant.

This chapter outlines some things you can do when you're actually pregnant to lower your risk of having another low-birthweight baby.

BEING A NON-SMOKER

One in three pregnant women smokes and the number of pregnant smokers is on the increase. Yet smoking is bad news for unborn babies (see p. 138 and p. 158) because not only may smoking damage your placenta – and the baby's supply of nutrients and oxygen – but each time you smoke, your baby does, too, which can lead to health problems after birth. The more you smoke, the more likely your baby is to be premature, and smoking more than 20 a day doubles the risk.

Cutting down is better than continuing to smoke a lot, but this still has dangers. For example, if you smoke up to nine cigarettes a day, your baby's risk of cot death in the first few months is twice that of a non-smoker's baby. And if you smoke ten or more, the risk is four times as high.

One survey found that only 41 per cent of pregnant smokers thought it important to cut down or stop, compared with 93 per cent of pregnant non-smokers. And according to the

Health Education Authority, only one in three pregnant smokers in the UK actually stopped in 1996. A few women say they continue because they want a small baby and therefore, they argue, an easier birth. The first part of this reasoning is logical, if foolish, because smoking retards a baby's growth. But a growth-retarded baby may have a very difficult birth. And she starts life with an increased risk of many health and development problems, both immediate, later in childhood, and in adult life.

So perhaps pregnant smokers either don't realise the very real dangers that accompany low birthweight, or need the stress-relief, relaxation and pleasure that come from smoking, and can think of no alternatives.

However, it's more valuable to stop smoking now than at any other time.

If you haven't yet stopped, don't forget that help is both available and successful (see Quitline, p. 178). But don't use nicotine patches as an aid because these aren't safe in pregnancy.

If you can't stop or choose not to, at least make sure you look after yourself and your baby by eating a healthy diet. And opt for middle-tar cigarettes, as low-tar varieties cause higher blood levels of carbon monoxide, a gas which reduces an unborn baby's oxygen supply.

EATING WELL

Eating well (see p. 134) in pregnancy is really important.

You'll probably put on 7–18kg (15–40lb). If after the first 12 weeks your weight doesn't increase as it should, you're probably not eating enough. Try not to miss a meal, but if you do, make up for it later.

Yet however careful you are it's difficult to eat well if money's tight, and some women give their partner and children enough to eat but go without themselves. This is bad for their health and their unborn baby's, too. If you'd like some tips on eating well, and on the benefits you can claim, NCH Action for Children (0171 226 2033) has a useful free leaflet, *Eating for Two on a Tight Budget*.

DRINKS

The Royal College of Obstetricians and Gynaecologists suggests pregnant women shouldn't drink alcohol. Department of Health experts say drinking no more than one or two units once or twice a week is unlikely to harm a baby. Whatever you do, it makes every sense to avoid getting drunk. Also, have no more than one or two cans of fizzy drinks a day.

EXERCISE

If you've had a premature baby before, or have reason to believe you might this time, avoid any contact sport or other exercise which could jar your body, such as jumping, jogging, high-impact aerobics – or even women's soccer.

SEX

Experts say gentle intercourse is unlikely to be harmful and there's no reason to abstain from sex.

If you've had one or more very premature labours before, then from 24 to 32 weeks (when prematurity is most risky), it might help for your partner to use a condom and you to avoid orgasm. I say this because, although never proved, there have been repeated suggestions that prostaglandins from semen at the cervix, or womb contractions from a woman's own orgasm, could – if the cervix is ripe and the womb primed – help trigger labour.

PRE-ECLAMPSIA

If you have pre-eclampsia or had it in a previous pregnancy, ask your doctor about a vitamin supplement (see p. 133). No benefit has yet been proved but it may help.

If you develop vision problems, a headache, stomach ache or unusual nausea, phone or see your doctor or midwife as you may need hospital admission.

TAKING ASPIRIN

If you have a high risk of having a premature baby, for example, because you've had one before, ask your doctor whether you should take aspirin each day. It's possible, though unproved, that a high daily dose (150mg) from very early pregnancy might help prevent pre-eclampsia in some high-risk women. However, studies show that 60mg daily has no effect on the risk of pre-eclampsia or pre-term birth.

If you've had several miscarriages (see Antiphospholipid Syndrome p. 139), ask your doctor about taking a low dose of aspirin a day. Trials suggest this makes some women less likely to miscarry and, presumably, less likely to have their baby prematurely.

VAGINAL DISCHARGE

See your doctor if you have an abnormal discharge in case you need treatment for an infection (see pp. 137 and 151).

SPECIAL CARE FOR TEETH AND GUMS

Gums are softer and more vulnerable to neglect in pregnancy – and some people find their teeth are too. You're entitled to free dental care at this time, so take advantage of it while you can. However, it's best to avoid having new amalgam (mercury-containing) fillings put in and old ones removed.

ITCHING

Report continued or severe itching to your doctor. Most pregnant women itch a little from time to time, but in a few this is a sign of a pregnancy-related liver disorder (obstetric cholestasis) which can lead to early labour.

TRAVEL

Take any medical information you have about your pregnancy when you travel, such as an antenatal clinic 'co-operation card'.

When in a car arrange the seatbelt so the diagonal strap lies between your breasts and the lower strap beneath your bump.

Going abroad? If you're expecting twins or more, or you've had a previous miscarriage, pre-term birth or low-birthweight baby, or you're likely to give birth early, it's best to travel only to places where you can rely on expert obstetric help.

IMMUNISATION

Remind your doctor you're pregnant when discussing travel immunisation. Live virus vaccines (including polio and yellow fever) are unsuitable and vaccines for other tropical diseases best avoided for three months before pregnancy.

INSURANCE

- You may have to pay a travel insurance premium in pregnancy.
- Take form E111 (from larger post offices) if travelling within the EC; this entitles you to free or part-free medical care, or allows reimbursement of some or all medical costs.
- If your destination is remote, make sure your insurance

covers MEDEVAC – a scheme enabling transport to a place where there's expert medical care.

FLYING

Most airlines don't accept pregnant women who are 35 weeks pregnant or more; some refuse after 28. It's wiser not to fly at all in the second half of pregnancy if you know you have a high risk of early labour.

PLANNED EARLY DELIVERY

If expecting a planned early delivery, you may like to ask the midwives if you can visit the SCBU to familiarise yourself with the layout and to meet the staff.

WORK

It's safe to work as long as you're fit and well, but if you've had one low-birthweight baby, it's best to avoid heavy physical work or standing for long periods.

If your work is very tiring or stressful, or if you work very long hours, it's best to give up or do something less onerous.

TELLING YOUR EMPLOYER

If your job could endanger you or the baby, it's best to inform your employer that you're pregnant as soon as possible so that your working conditions can be monitored or altered, or your role changed. Potentially hazardous activities include working with ionising radiation and certain chemicals. You are entitled to alternative work if necessary for your safety.

If you have any questions about employment rights, ring the Maternity Alliance helpline (see p. 177) or request its leaflet, *Sickness, Pregnancy and Maternity Leave – Your Employment Rights*.

MATERNITY PAY AND BENEFITS

Information about maternity pay and benefits is available from:

- Your employer
- Your benefits agency
- The free leaflet, *Babies and Benefits*, from the Department of Social Security, Leaflets Unit, PO Box 21, Stanmore, Middlesex HA7 1AY
- The leaflet, *Pregnant at Work*: send £1 plus an sae to the Maternity Alliance (see p. 177).

All these try to make the information clear – but it is complicated, so if you don't understand, go on asking until you're satisfied.

'RECREATIONAL' DRUGS

If – against all advice – you're still using drugs, ask friends who've been pregnant, or your midwife, health visitor or doctor, if they know of any special facilities for women who are pregnant and on drugs. Some areas have a special antenatal discussion group, class or clinic where the staff will have a particular interest in making you feel comfortable and giving you the information you need.

RELAXATION

You are doing an extremely important thing by carrying a baby and you need plenty of time to relax. So don't push yourself too hard, but take time each day to do absolutely nothing with your feet up. You and your baby will both reap a lot of benefits if you care for you both in this way.

Finally, we'll look at antenatal care.

CHAPTER 18

Antenatal Care, Tests and Treatment

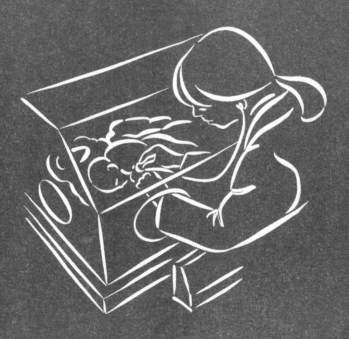

Antenatal care can reduce your risk of having another low-birthweight baby, enable planned early delivery, if necessary, at the best time, and familiarise the doctors with your situation so they save valuable time deciding what to do if you go into premature labour.

WHERE TO GO

Make an early appointment with your doctor. You're legally entitled to time off work to visit the antenatal clinic and for parentcraft classes.

Your doctor will recommend a folic acid and, perhaps, other supplements (see pp. 147–148), and check you aren't taking drugs which might harm the baby. He may, with a midwife's help, provide some antenatal care or suggest you have it all at hospital. As you've had a premature baby before, you have a higher risk of having one this time, too (see p. 139), so he'll probably recommend a hospital birth.

Some women have a raised risk of having a low-birthweight baby, yet don't like visiting the doctor's surgery or hospital. Fortunately, some areas have:

'**Drop-in centres**', where appointments are unnecessary, for:
• Teenage girls
• Homeless women
• Drug users.

Community centre clinics or other facilities for women who may need antenatal care offered in a particular way, for example:

- Those from Asian or other ethnic communities with little English
- Those whose culture means the antenatal information they receive needs a different slant
- Those whose partners don't want them seeing a male doctor
- Those with a learning or other disability.

ANTENATAL CLINIC VISITS

Many women have their first hospital check – the 'booking visit' – at around 12 weeks and 15 scheduled antenatal checks altogether, but you may be asked to attend more often.

ROUTINE MEASUREMENTS AND TESTS

Your doctor or midwife will check:

- **Your blood pressure** (see p. 132)
- **Your urine for glucose**, a possible, though unreliable, sign of diabetes (see p. 136). A blood sugar test after a glucose drink is more accurate for suspected diabetes. Your urine may also be checked for protein (a possible sign of pre-eclampsia and urine infection)
- **The growth of your womb and baby**. At the first visit the staff will weigh you and work out your BMI (body mass index – weight in kilograms divided by height in metres squared). If abnormally low, then unless you go on to have a good weight gain (see p. 134), your baby may have a low birth-weight. You may be weighed each time. The doctor or midwife will feel your abdomen and may offer one or more screening tests to check the baby's growth and development

- **Your baby's heartbeat**. The midwife or doctor will listen to his heart with a metal trumpet called a fetal stethoscope or a hand-held ultrasound device
- **Your blood**, for your blood group and rhesus factor, anaemia, rubella immunity, and infection (including hepatitis B and syphilis). Some antenatal clinics test for toxoplasmosis and HIV infections. You'll be screened for sickle cell disease if you are of Afro-Caribbean descent, and for thalassaemia if you are of Asian or Mediterranean descent.

ANTENATAL CLASSES

Once you are more than eight weeks pregnant, ask your midwife about NHS antenatal classes, or find the number of your local NCT (National Childbirth Trust) teacher and ask about her classes. Sometimes classes or discussion groups are available at drop-in centres and local community centres (see above). And midwives in at least one hospital (Southend) run a special weekly group for pregnant women under 20.

Antenatal teachers provide information about pregnancy and birth, offer discussion, and teach muscle relaxation and breathing control for use in labour. Antenatal classes are also a good place to make new friends.

YOUR BIRTH PLAN

You may like to plan how you'd ideally like labour conducted – whether or not you give birth prematurely or have complications. Making a plan clarifies ideas and guides your birth attendants as to how you think you'd like to be helped and, if necessary, treated.

But a birth plan is not a set of rules because no one knows what will happen, so it's wise to couch it in terms of 'if possible' and 'ideally'.

SPECIAL TESTS AND PROCEDURES

Some women are offered a fetal fibronectin test (see p. 173) and a test for vaginal infection (see p. 151) to assess their risk of delivering prematurely.

Ultrasound scans can help track a baby's progress, and these and maternal serum screening can detect a raised risk of malformations and genetic abnormalities, some of which lead to a low birthweight.

Screening tests are offered early so that if they suggest that a more accurate test is necessary, and this reveals an abnormality, a woman can consider abortion.

WHY BE SCREENED IF YOU WOULDN'T HAVE AN ABORTION?

Many doctors believe screening tests are worthwhile even for a woman who disagrees with abortion, because knowing her baby has an abnormality gives her and her partner time to get used to the idea and to prepare to welcome their baby. However, I think many doctors realise that a woman confronted with the reality of carrying an abnormal baby is likely to change her mind about abortion. Most women in this situation decide on abortion, however sadly and reluctantly.

If you want to know more about the purpose, accuracy, side effects and implications of any test or procedure – or if you're upset about anything – make time to discuss your concerns with your doctor or midwife.

ULTRASOUND SCANNING

In the UK 95 per cent of women have one or more scans

During a scan a technician slides a probe emitting high-frequency sound waves over your abdomen. Sound reflected from the baby is transformed into an image on a TV screen.

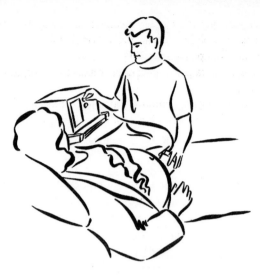

Sometimes the probe gives a clearer image if placed in the vagina. Your baby may move around more during a scan.

Most doctors believe scans are safe and claim that even if a risk were ever proven, the advantages would far outweigh it.

The most common times for a scan are at:

10–14 *weeks*: confirms whether your baby's size matches your dates, and picks up multiple pregnancy and about 70 per cent of major structural abnormalities (including anencephaly – a fatal skull and brain defect – and spina bifida – a spine and spinal cord defect).

18–20 *weeks*: an ordinary scan detects most structural malformations and shows the placenta's size and position. A Doppler scan can detect a reduced blood flow in the womb and umbilical arteries, indicating a higher chance of pre-eclampsia, growth-retardation, or both.

You may have a scan at other times to check whether:
• You have miscarried (after bleeding from the womb)

- The pregnancy is ectopic (meaning the baby is growing outside the womb) – usually in a Fallopian tube
- Your cervix is ripe (see p. 130)
- There's placenta praevia – a dangerously low-lying placenta (see p. 136)
- Your baby is big and mature enough to be born
- Your baby is in the breech position.

MATERNAL SERUM SCREENING

Many hospitals offer serum screening for major abnormalities at 15–20 weeks. An ultrasound scan first confirms the baby's age. Serum screening detects up to four out of five Down's babies and indicates a high risk of spina bifida. But false positives and negatives are possible.

The double, triple and quadruple tests measure the levels of two, three or four markers (alpha-fetoprotein, chorionic gonadotrophin, oestriol and inhibin A) in the mother's blood. The risk of abnormality is estimated from the result and from the woman's age. The quadruple test is the most reliable.

Researchers are studying whether a test of fetal DNA (genetic material) in the mother's blood – present in four in five women – should replace amniocentesis; they think this may be reliable as early as 11 weeks. Others are assessing a test of HCG (human chorionic gonadotrophin) and pregnancy-associated protein A, which can be done at 10–14 weeks.

A high-risk, 'positive' screening test result means you'll be offered a procedure enabling a more accurate test for chromosome abnormalities (such as Down's syndrome and sickle cell disease). If this reveals an abnormality, your doctor will offer an abortion.

A risk of one or more in 250 of a baby being affected is considered high or positive. It *also indicates a 249 in 250 chance of the baby not being affected.*

PROCEDURES ENABLING ACCURATE TESTS FOR CHROMOSOMAL ABNORMALITIES

These include chorionic villus sampling, amniocentesis and fetal blood sampling. Each produces fetal cells for chromosome culture. And each carries a risk to the baby.

CHORIONIC VILLUS SAMPLING (CVS)

You may be offered sampling and testing of placental cells at 11–12 weeks. Guided by real-time ultrasound scanning, the doctor puts a needle through the woman's abdomen into the placenta and sucks out some cells. Chromosomes are karyotyped ('cultured' or grown) and examined for genetic problems. The result is available in one to two weeks. Sometimes repeat testing is necessary. Occasionally a sample of the placenta is taken through the cervix.

One or two babies in 100 dies after CVS.

AMNIOCENTESIS

Some hospitals routinely offer amniocentesis at 14–18 weeks to women with a raised risk of an abnormal baby. Guided by a real-time ultrasound scan, the doctor takes a sample of fluid from around the baby through a needle passed through the woman's abdomen into the womb. Chromosomes from the baby's cells in the fluid are karyotyped and examined for genetic problems. The result is available within three weeks.

An 'amnio' isn't always straightforward:
- The needle occasionally damages the baby
- One in 100 babies dies afterwards
- Chromosomes fail to grow three times in 1000.

FETAL BLOOD SAMPLING (CORDOCENTESIS)

In some units a baby's blood is sampled after 18 weeks if there's a risk of an infection such as rubella or toxoplasmosis.

It can also be used to examine chromosomes. Guided by a real-time ultrasound scan the doctor puts a needle through the woman's abdomen into her womb, and into the baby's umbilical vein.

One or two in every 100 babies dies afterwards.

GENETIC COUNSELLING

If you've had a baby with a genetic abnormality or have a family history of a genetic disorder, genetic counselling can help you decide whether to have tests. Your doctor can give you more information.

FETAL FIBRONECTIN TEST (see p. 7)

The fetal fibronectin test – under evaluation by the PREMET trial and available only in south-east London at the time of writing – indicates whether pre-term labour is likely. It's useful for a woman who:

- May be in early labour (see p. 2)
- Has had a premature birth before
- Has a raised risk of premature labour because of too much fluid in the womb (see p. 140)
- Is carrying twins or more.

Swabs of vaginal mucus are tested for fetal fibronectin at 24 and 27 weeks. Its presence after 20 weeks indicates a one in five chance of premature labour within four weeks.

BACTERIAL INFECTION OR OVER-GROWTH TEST

The doctor may arrange for vaginal swabs to be tested for bacterial infection or overgrowth (see p. 137).

KICK COUNT

If your baby is growing too slowly, your doctor may ask you to record movements. In the last few months of pregnancy there are generally ten or more kicks in 12 hours. Few or no kicks may indicate something wrong and lead to emergency delivery.

HORMONE TESTS

Blood tests for oestriol or placental lactogen indicate how well your placenta is performing and may be done if your baby seems unusually small.

PREVIOUS MISCARRIAGES OR PREMATURE LABOURS

If you've had several miscarriages, your doctor may do a blood test for antiphospholipid syndrome (see p. 139). Pre-eclampsia (see p. 132) is another possible cause.

Your doctor may recommend aspirin if you have one of these.

PREVENTING RHESUS DISEASE

If your blood group is rhesus-negative, your doctor may give you injections of anti-D immunoglobulin (see p. 45) at 28 and 34 weeks. This prevents you developing antibodies which could destroy the red blood cells in any future rhesus-positive babies you may have. This condition is called rhesus disease. It's also advisable if you have a threatened miscarriage with heavy or repeated bleeding or pain.

TREATING FETAL ILLNESS IN THE WOMB

Some illnesses are managed in the womb to prevent early delivery becoming necessary. Severe rhesus disease, for example, can be treated by intra-uterine transfusion.

THE FUTURE FOR SURROGATE MOTHERS AND ARTIFICIAL WOMBS

Some women can't grow a baby big enough or carry one long enough to survive. Already such a woman can arrange for a surrogate mother to carry her baby. The surrogate's womb is primed by hormone treatment. A doctor adds the father's sperm to the mother's egg in a test tube. Then the resulting embryo is put in the surrogate's womb.

Researchers are applying their minds to the possibility of ventilating extremely premature babies with a perfluorocarbon oil which easily takes up oxygen and carbon dioxide. They hope this might prevent lung damage from early and prolonged ventilation. One day advances such as this may even make it possible to grow a baby in an artificial womb!

HELP LIST

ORGANISATIONS

Action for Pre-Eclampsia (APEC)
31–33 College Road
Harrow
Middlesex HA1 1EJ
Tel: 0181 427 4217

Active Birth Centre
113a Chetwynd Road
London NW5 1DA
Tel: 0171 482 5554

Association for Postnatal Illness
25 Jerdan Place
London SW6 1BE
Tel: 0171 386 0868

BLISS (Baby Life Support Systems)
17–21 Emerald Street
London WC1N 3QL
Tel: 0171 831 9393/8996
Freephone helpline: 0500 618 140
(Sponsors SCBU equipment and neonatal nurse training)

Blisslink/Nippers – address as for BLISS.

Free helpline: 0500 618 140
(Information; support for parents of premature and special-care babies from 'befrienders' who have them-selves had a special-care baby; penfriend scheme; 'home on oxygen' information; 'Special Memories' bereavement group (with a newsletter, befrienders' register and local support groups); links with other parent support groups; newsletter)

Breast-milk bank guidelines
(for health professionals) are available from:
British Paediatric Association
50 Hallam Street
London W1N 6DE

The Child Bereavement Trust
Harleyford Estate
Henley Road, Marlow
Buckinghamshire SL7 2DX
Tel: 01628 488 101
(Books, tapes and videos to guide adults and children through their loss; training of professional carers in support-ing and counselling)

Contact a Family
170 Tottenham Court Road
London W1P 0HA
Tel: 0171 383 3555
(Has a register of support organisations for parents of children with nearly every common and rare condition)

CRY-SIS
BM Cry-sis
London WC1N 3XX
Helpline: 0171 404 5011
(Help and support if your baby cries a lot)

Foresight Charity for Preconceptual Care
28 The Paddock
Godalming
Surrey GU7 1XD
Tel: 01483 427839
(Information about preconceptual care)

Foundation for the Study of Infant Deaths
14 Halkin Street
London SW1X 7DP
Helpline: 0171 235 1721
(Support and information after a cot death)

Homestart UK
2 Salisbury Road
Leicester LE1 7QR
Tel: 0116 233 9955
(Befriender support for parents of under-fives)

(Volunteers offer support and practical help)

La Leche League
BM 3424
London WC1N 3XX
Tel: 0171 242 1278
Website: http:// www.laleche-league.org/
(Breastfeeding support and information)

The Maternity Alliance
45 Beech Street
London EC2P 2LX
(Campaigns for rights and services for families, offers leaflets, booklets and other publications, and has a maternity rights helpline on 0171 588 8582)

Meet-a-Mum Association (MAMA)
26 Avenue Road
South Norwood
London SE25 4EX
Tel: 0181 771 5595
(Offers contacts for all mothers and support for postnatal depression)

National Childbirth Trust
Alexandra House
Oldham Terrace
London W3 6NH
Tel: 0181 992 8637
(Offers antenatal classes and postnatal support)

National Childbirth Trust (Maternity Sales) Ltd
Catalogue from:
239 Shawbridge Street
Glasgow G43 1QN
Tel: 0141 636 0600

Parentline
Tel: 01702 559 900
(For counselling when under stress)

The Parent Network
Room 2
Winchester House
11 Cranmer Road
London SW9 6EJ
Tel: 0171 735 1214
(Support and education for parents)

Quitline
Tel: 0800 00 22 00
(For help to stop smoking. A pregnancy Quitline – 0800 00 22 11 – currently operating in the Doncaster area may become nationally available)

SPARKS (SPort Aiding Medical Research for KidS)
Francis House
Francis Street
London SW1P 1DE
Tel: 0171 931 8899
(Fundraising for research into low birthweight)

Stillbirth and Neonatal Death Society (SANDS)
28 Portland Place
London W1N 4DE
Tel: 0171 436 5881
(Offers support)

Tommy's Campaign
1 Kennington Road
London SE1 7RR
Tel: 0171 620 0188
(Funds research into premature birth, miscarriage and stillbirth)

Twins and Multiple Birth Association (TAMBA)
Harnott House
309 Chester Road
Little Sutton
South Wirral
Merseyside L66 1QQ
Tel: 0151 348 0020

UK Baby Friendly Initiative
20 Guilford Street
London WC1N 1DZ
(Makes awards to hospitals which facilitate breastfeeding)

Women's Aid National Helpline
Tel: 0345 023 468

BOOKS AND LEAFLETS

Breastfeeding Special Care Babies by Sandra Lang (Baillière Tindall)

Breast Is Best by Drs Penny and Andrew Stanway (Pan)

Easy Exercises for Pregnancy by Janet Balaskas (Frances Lincoln)

How to Remove Old Lead Paint (leaflet available from Paintmakers Association, James House, Bridge Street, Leatherhead, Surrey KT22 7EP, Tel: 01372 360 660)

Kangaroo Care by Kathy Sleath (available from BLISS, see above)

Massage for the Newborn Needing Special Care by Cherry Bond (send sae for mail-order details to the SCBU, Queen Charlotte's and Chelsea Hospital, Goldhawk Road, London W6 0XG)

Milk Banking: News and Views (newsletter available from Gillian Weaver, Human Milk Bank, Queen Charlotte's and Chelsea Hospital, Goldhawk Road, London W6 0XG)

The Mothercare New Guide to Pregnancy and Babycare edited by Dr Penny Stanway (Conran Octopus)

My Book about Our Baby Who Died by Lynda Weiss and Jenni Thomas (available from the Child Bereavement Trust, see above) – a workbook for children aged three to ten

Poor Expectations: Poverty and Undernourishment in Pregnancy by Julie Dallison and Tim Lobstein (NCH Action for Children and The Maternity Alliance)

Special Care Babies by Althea (available from Blisslink/Nippers, see above) – explains special care to children

This Is Your Baby (send sae for mail-order details to Margaret Sparshott, SCBU, Plymouth General Hospital, Freedom Fields, Plymouth, Devon PL4 8QQ)

PRODUCTS

Baby clothes: the following companies sell clothes for small babies:

Babycare-Dollycare (Cosby) Ltd
2 Winchester Avenue
Blaby Bypass
Blaby
Leicester LE8 4GZ
Tel: 0116 278 3336

BLISS (see p. 176) has knitting patterns.

Small Wonders
PO Box 13
Newport TF10 7WS

Tiddlywinks
Moorland House
3 Willow Tree Gardens
Eldwick
Bingley BD16 3HN
Tel: 01274 561 751

Breast pumps: to rent or buy from The National Childbirth Trust (see above); La Leche League (see above); Ameda-Egnell Ltd, Unit 1, Belvedere Trading Estate, Taunton, Somerset TA1 1BH, Tel: 01823 336 362; smaller hand pumps to order from pharmacies and medical supply shops.

Car seats: adjustable for low-birthweight babies from Bettacare Ltd, 9-10 Faygate Business Centre, Faygate, West Sussex RH12 4DN Tel: 01293 851 896

Food Supplements: suitable when waiting to conceive and during pregnancy, from pharmacies and other retail outlets. Examples of multivita-min and mineral supplements include Pregnacare (Vitabiotics), Pregnancy (Boots), PreNatal Formula (General Nutrition Centres) and Pregnancy Pack (Health Plus). An example of an essential fatty acid supplement is Efanatal (Efamol Ltd).

Nappies: Boots sell 'pre-mini' nappies for up to 3000g (6lb); Pampers do 'micro-nappies' for over 1000g (2lb).

Slings: from 2500g (4lb 14oz) upwards from Wilkinet Baby Carrier, PO Box 20, Cardigan, Wales SA43 1JB, Tel: 01239 841 844

Supplementer: available from Central Medical Supplies, CMS House, Basford Lane, Leek Brook, Leek, Staffordshire, ST13 7DT. Tel: 01538 399 541 *also available from*

THE ORION PUBLISHING GROUP

Apples & Pears £3.99
GLORIA THOMAS
0 75281 604 7

Are You Getting Enough?
£4.99
ANGELA DOWDEN
0 75281 702 7

Arousing Aromas £3.99
KAY COOPER
0 75281 546 6

Body Foods For Women
£6.99
JANE CLARKE
0 75280 922 9

Cranks Recipe Book £6.99
CRANKS RESTAURANTS
1 85797 140 X

Eat Safely £3.99
JANET WRIGHT
0 75281 544 X

Entertaining with
Cranks £6.99
CRANKS RESTAURANTS
0 75282 579 8

Food £6.99
SUSAN POWTER
0 75280 315 8

The Good Mood Guide
£4.99
ROS & JEREMY HOLMES
0 75282 584 4

Harmonise Your Home
£4.99
GRAHAM GUNN
0 75281 665 9

Health Spa at Home £3.99
JOSEPHINE FAIRLEY
0 75281 545 8

Juice Up Your Energy Levels
£3.99
LESLEY WATERS
0 75281 602 0

Kitchen Pharmacy £7.99
ROSE ELLIOT & CARLO DE
PAOLI
0 75281 725 6

A Natural History
of the Senses £7.99
DIANE ACKERMAN
1 85799 403 5

The Natural Way To Stop
Snoring £4.99
DR. ELIZABETH SCOTT
0 75280 067 1

The New Cranks Recipe
Book £6.99
NADINE ABENSUR
0 75281 677 2

Sensitive Skin £4.99
JOSEPHINE FAIRLEY
0 75281 547 4

Spring Clean Your System
JANE GARTON £3.99
0 75281 601 2

Stop the Insanity! £6.99
SUSAN POWTER
1 85797 323 2

Vegetarian Slimming £6.99
ROSE ELLIOT
0 75280 173 2

All Orion/Phoenix titles are available at your local bookshop or from the following address:

Littlehampton Book Services
Cash Sales Department L
14 Eldon Way, Lineside Industrial Estate
Littlehampton
West Sussex BN17 7HE

telephone 01903 721596, *facsimile* 01903 730914

Payment can either be made by credit card (Visa and Mastercard accepted) or by sending a cheque or postal order made payable to *Littlehampton Book Services*.

DO NOT SEND CASH OR CURRENCY.

Please add the following to cover postage and packing

UK and BFPO:
£1.50 for the first book, and 50p for each additional book to a maximum of £3.50

Overseas and Eire:
£2.50 for the first book plus £1.00 for the second book and 50p for each additional book ordered

---

BLOCK CAPITALS PLEASE

name of cardholder ....

delivery address
(if different from cardholder)

address of cardholder ....

....

....

....

postcode ....

postcode ....

☐ I enclose my remittance for £.............................

☐ please debit my Mastercard/Visa (delete as appropriate)

card number ☐☐☐☐☐☐☐☐☐☐☐☐☐☐☐☐☐☐

expiry date ☐☐☐☐

signature ....

prices and availability are subject to change without notice